Damaged Goods?

Damaged Goods?

Women Living with Incurable
Sexually Transmitted Diseases

Adina Nack

TEMPLE UNIVERSITY PRESS
Philadelphia

Earlier versions of material in Chapters 1, 4, and 8 appeared in "Bad Girls and Fallen Women: Chronic STD Diagnoses as Gateways to Tribal Stigma," 25(4): 463-485, ©2002 by *Symbolic Interaction*. Earlier versions of material in chapters 1, 5, and 8 appeared in "Damaged Goods: Women Managing the Stigma of STDs," (21): 95-121, ©2000 by *Deviant Behavior.*

Temple University Press
1601 North Broad Street
Philadelphia PA 19122
www.temple.edu/tempress

∞ The paper used in this publication meets the requirements
of the American National Standard for Information Sciences—Permanence of Paper
for Printed Library Materials, ANSI Z39.48-1992

Library of Congress Cataloging-in-Publication Data

Nack, Adina, 1972–
    Damaged goods? Women living with incurable sexually transmitted
diseases / Adina Nack.
        p. ; cm.
    Includes bibliographical references and index.
    ISBN-13: 978-1-59213-707-7 (cloth : alk. paper)
    ISBN-13: 978-1-59213-708-4 (pbk. : alk. paper)
    ISBN-10: 1-59213-707-5 (cloth : alk. paper)
    ISBN-10: 1-59213-708-3 (pbk. : alk. paper)   1. Sexually transmitted
diseases—Social aspects.   2. Women—Diseases—Social aspects.   3. Papillomavirus
diseases—Social aspects.   4. Herpes genitalis—Social aspects.   I. Title.
    [DNLM: 1. Sexually Transmitted Diseases—psychology—
United States.   2. Chronic Disease—psychology—United States.   3. Morals—
United States.   4. Sexual Behavior—United States.   5. Women—United States.
WC 140 N125d 2008]
    RA644.V4N33 2008
    362.196'951—dc22   2007050273

2   4   6   8   9   7   5   3   1

For the unnamed millions who live with
incurable sexually transmitted diseases.
May we all soon live in a world where no one views you
as damaged goods.

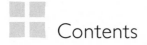

Contents

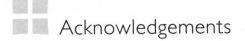

Acknowledgements

Without the support—personal, intellectual, and financial—of my family and family of friends, this book would have never been completed. Many friends and extended family members have stood by me throughout the years of my illness and this project, including: Carolyn Aibel, Graziella Awabdy, Judy Ball, Bobby Eghbalieh, Suki Fisher, Adam Griff, Dave Horwitz, Jen Kam, Marie Lyons, Rujuta Manghani, Natasha Tolstikova, Jen Vineyard, and Rachel Wilson. I cannot thank my parents enough—Susan and Myron Nack, who encouraged me throughout the traumas of my own HPV experiences, during the trials and tribulations of my graduate school years, and the stress of my early years in academia. Thanks to my sister, Jaime Nack, for being so supportive of this research. Thanks to my in-laws, Frank and Manuela Marichal, for their love and support, and for never being ashamed that their son married a woman who has been so public about having an STD, being a sexual health researcher and an activist. Special thanks to my husband, José Marichal, for being my life partner—in every sense of the word—and never letting me doubt my ability to complete the research and to write this book. I thank God for giving José and I the gift of our daughter, Hana, who, not only confirmed that I was not so "damaged" by HPV, but also fills everyday of my life with joy and wonder.

This book began as a doctoral dissertation at the University of Colorado, Boulder. I am indebted to the hands-on guidance from my advisor, Patti Adler, and to my incredibly helpful co-advisor, Peter Adler. Many thanks also to Lerita Coleman, Leslie Irvine, Alison Jaggar, Joyce Nielsen, and David Pellow for being active members of my dissertation committee and believing in my work early on. I also am grateful to fellow grad students, who made up our 'dissertation support group,' and helped me throughout the research process: Alice Fothergill, Katy Irwin, and Jen Lois. I could not have asked for more wonderful grad school friends and especially want to thank Matt Brown, Kris De Welde, Carrie Foote, Stacy Mallicoat, Linda Ramos, Elisabeth Sheff, and Glenda Walden. I also appreciate the professional opportunities and research support afforded to me by the staff of the Community Health Education Department and Women's Health Clinic at the University of Colorado's Wardenburg Health Center.

I would like to express my thanks to my first colleagues at the University of Maine for believing in my future as a medical sociologist: Especially to Steve Barkan, Leslie King, and Stephen Marks, for their encouragement of my early writing about this research. During my final years of writing, I relocated to California Lutheran University, and I am very appreciative of the affirmation and support given to me by Michael Brint, Jonathan Cordero, Pat Egle, Greg Freeland, Charles Hall, Tim Hengst, Cindy Jew, Ken Kambara, Chris Kimball, Marja Mogk, Nandra Perry, Mindy Puopolo, Gail Uellendahl, Akiko Yasuike, and, in the 'homestretch,' my undergraduate assistant, Cheyanne Anderson.

For the many generous sources of financial support that I received toward the completion of my doctoral work, I wish to thank the University of Colorado's Graduate School for a fellowship and a grant, as well as the Boulder, Colorado branch of the American Association of University Women for a grant. I also gratefully acknowledge the 2000 Graduate Student Paper Award presented to me by Health, Health Policy, and Health Services Division of the Society for the Study of Social Problems, which motivated me to complete my dissertation. I was honored by the 2001 Herbert Blumer Award, granted to me by the Society for the Study of Symbolic Interaction, which encouraged me to revise my dissertation into this book.

My sincere gratitude to Janet Fancendese and Temple University Press for giving me the opportunity to revise and expand my previous work. Janet has been an incredibly supportive editor, and I am grateful for the anonymous reviewers, whose comments have inspired and challenged my thinking about women's sexual health.

Finally, I thank the forty-three women who trusted me with their stories. I hope that each one of them can see how much they have influenced my work and, hopefully, made a positive difference in the lives of others, who may feel alone in their STD struggles.

Mixing Morality with Medicine

I never thought it would happen to me . . .

A 20-year-old undergraduate receives a phone call from her ex-boyfriend. He nervously informs her that he has just been diagnosed with genital warts and is in the process of having them "frozen off" with liquid nitrogen. He explains that he called her because there was a chance that he might have had *this* when they had last *been together*. He adds that he is not sure she is at risk because he had not noticed symptoms until recently. She quickly thanks him for calling, hangs up the phone, and sits in stunned silence.

She thinks to herself: *How could this have happened to me? I'm not a slut: I've only had sex with three guys and always used condoms. I talked with both my ex-boyfriends and current boyfriend before we ever had sex—they told me about their sexual histories and sexual health. These guys had all tested negative for HIV, so they were "safe"—healthy and trustworthy—right? My high school sex education focused on HIV/AIDS, so I've only been worried about fluids being transmitted. Is it possible to get a disease even when you're using condoms?*

A series of scary questions runs through her mind. *Do I have warts, too? How could I? My last annual gynecological exam was less than six months ago, and my Pap smear results were normal. Wouldn't my doctor have noticed if I had warts? Could I have warts that are so tiny I've never noticed them? Have I already infected my current boy-friend?*

With no answers to any of these questions, one horrific image ap-pears in her mind with unsettling clarity: inspired by the one film about sexually transmitted diseases (STDs[1]) that was shown in her high school health class, she envisions her vulva sprouting cauliflower-like growths, more and more fleshy warts, ultimately covering her genitals inside and out. This image brings her to tears. As she begins to cry, she wonders: *Will any guy ever want me? Will I ever get married or be able to have a healthy baby?*[2]

More than Just an Infection: Gendered Morality and Sexual Diseases

The preceding snapshot gives one example of how it feels to find out that you have a STD. Many infected individuals feel "dirty," disgusted by the bumps and sores that require medical attention and mar body parts, which are supposed to be the most private, sensual, and erotic. These negative feelings are compounded by the social acceptability of blaming infected individuals for their illnesses. Often the blame comes with judgments, such as *irresponsible, naïve,* or *stupid*. Others will likely view this illness as a sign of immorality and label the infected person a promiscuous *slut*, having low character and bad values. This kind of disease will likely be experienced not only as a health crisis but also as an identity crisis. It is easy to understand why many Americans with STDs are left wondering if they are, in fact, *damaged goods*—their bodies and reputations so spoiled that they may never again feel healthy, whole, and valuable.

Every year, versions of this scenario become reality for many of the over 15 million Americans who contract a STD. Chronic STDs are a significant part of this epidemic in the sexually-active popula-tion: U.S. rates of genital human papillomavirus[3] infections (HPV—the virus that causes anogenital warts and cervical lesions) are as high as 75 percent (ASHA 2006a), and genital herpes infections (HSV) are estimated at more than 20 percent (ASHA 2006b). Since 2000, HPV infection has ranked as the most common STD infecting American youth (Weinstock et al. 2004). Medical experts believe that these rates will continue to rise, in part because genital HSV and HPV infections are often asymptomatic and frequently transmitted by individuals who do not know that they are infected. If present, symptoms may be mild, mistaken for other conditions, or seem to be "cured" during long periods of latency.[4] The failure to recognize symptoms of these infections translates into a serious public health problem because both of these viruses are contagious, even in the absence of noticeable symptoms.

A recent study pointed out that, "[w]hile these diseases are of epidemic proportion, we actually see surprising little about them in the media, and we talk about them even less" (Cline 2006:353). In an era of public health campaigns and mandated education targeting HIV/AIDS, the use of latex condoms is more and more the behavioral norm for "safer" sex. However, both HPV and HSV are transmitted by skin-to-skin contact.[5] So, even when a latex condom is used consistently and correctly, it will provide a barrier for only a portion of the genital skin that will likely come in contact with a partner's skin during sexual intercourse. In addition to the promotion of using latex condoms as the standard for 'safer sex,' HIV-testing has also been successfully promoted as a sexual responsibility norm. Currently, more than 50 percent of adults have only been tested for HIV and not for any other STDs (ASHA 2006c). Given our medical norm of annual gynecological exams for women, but no comparable exam for men, a significant portion of the sexually-active population is not regularly screened for any STDs.

When individuals do seek sexual health exams, less than one-third of US physicians consistently screen these patients for the full range of sexually transmitted diseases, leaving many patients unaware of their infection status with regard to either HPV or HSV (ASHA 2006c).[6] Some sexual health educators believe that, because these two diseases are understood as nonfatal, there has been less funding for research, education, and prevention efforts. However, genital herpes and HPV infections can have devastating effects if transferred from mother to fetus, and medical researchers have linked certain strains of HPV to cervical and anal cancers.[7]

Odds are, you have not heard of the "HPV vaccine." On the other hand, if you live in the U.S., then you have probably seen or heard one of many ads promoting a "cervical cancer" vaccine sold by Merck as

GARDASIL. Originally, this vaccine was called what it actually is: a vaccine to protect against several strains of sexually transmitted human papillomavirus (HPV). When the press began to cover the trials of this HPV vaccine, several conservative organizations protested. The Family Research Council (FRC), for example, was initially concerned that the HPV vaccine equated to a "license" for young people to have premarital sex. Strong objections from such socially-conservative organizations, in addition to focus groups conducted by the CDC, may have informed Merck's marketing campaign of GARDASIL, in which all advertisements, marketing, and health education materials aim to sell this to the American public as a vaccine that protects against cervical cancer. Parry (2007) notes that this is not an easy plan or necessarily a solution to the problem of longstanding negative stigma against STDs: "Promoting an anti-cancer vaccine and, at the same time, making it clear that HPV is a sexually transmitted infection will require deft handling in the wording of policy, education and publicity materials" (90). Many health organizations, including the American Cancer Society, expressed concerns that acceptance of the drug would be influenced by whether the American public perceives the vaccine to be one aimed at reducing the risk of cervical cancer, or as a vaccine designed to prevent a sexually transmitted virus.

So, is there really a "cervical cancer" vaccine? In short, the answer is "No." Merck's vaccine, trademarked as GARDASIL, protects against four HPV types, which together are associated with 70 percent of cervical cancers, but these cancers are relatively rare. The American Cancer Society estimated that, in 2006, approximately 9,710 women were diagnosed with invasive cervical cancer and another 3,700 died from it (2007). In June 2006, the Food and Drug Administration (FDA) licensed GARDASIL, a prophylactic vaccine[8], that prevents over 95 percent of HPV infections, caused by four types of virus: Together, these are estimated to be responsible for about 70 percent of cervical cancers (HPV types 16 and 18) and 90 percent of genital warts (HPV types 6 and 11) (Temte 2007). This vaccine is not an effective treatment for existing HPV infections (genital warts, cervical cancers or precancerous lesions). It has been tested and approved for use on girls and women from 9 to 26 years of age. Given the expense, limitations, and controversies surrounding this new approach to the prevention of HPV, the ultimate impact of this vaccine remains to be seen. As this new vaccine protects against only four strains of HPV, girls and women who receive the vaccine will need to continue routine gynecological exams and practice safer sexual behaviors[9], as these individuals will be vulnerable to infection with the dozen or so other strains of this virus. As for the ongoing work on developing an HSV (herpes) vaccine, medical researchers are not sure whether a safe and effective one will be developed. Those who study pediatric infectious diseases have noted that, "Once an efficacious herpes vaccine is available, its effectiveness will depend ultimately on vaccine acceptance by professional organizations, healthcare professionals, and parents" (Rupp et al. 2005, 31).

The development and widespread use of any STD vaccines will not necessarily result in a world that is kinder and gentler to those who become infected. In fact, there is reason to believe that STD-related stigma may negatively affect the public's response to the new vaccine that is being marketed as a "cervical cancer" vaccine. A recent behavioral health article on HPV and cervical cancer emphasized the need for research that explores how the nature of this virus being sexually-transmitted affects the experiences of those who test positive. These findings could help us to better understand how individuals will make decisions about cervical cancer screening (Waller et al.2004) (See Chapter 8 for more discussion of STD vaccines.).

The cost of diagnosing and treating all sexually transmitted diseases in the U.S. is about $8 billion per year. HPV and HSV account for a sizeable portion of these costs (ASHA 2006c): HPV infections alone add up to health care expenses of over $2 billion per year (CDC 2006). It is difficult, however, to put a price tag on the variety of personal costs to infected individuals. Individuals experience social and psychological costs of these infections differently, depending upon their sex, socioeconomic status, ethnicity, age, religious upbringing, and other factors. Sex differences are the most obvious: HPV and HSV present more negative consequences for women, in terms of both reproductive health and self-concept. For instance, a woman's reproductive health can be greatly compromised by a cervical HPV infection that necessitates the removal of significant amounts of her cervix, the bottom portion of the uterus, which must be thick enough and strong enough to bear the weight of a growing fetus. Should she be able to carry the baby to term, there is the additional risk that, genital infections of both HPV and HSV can pass from mothers to babies during vaginal deliveries.

Although the CDC reports that few women suffer serious reproductive consequences of HPV and HSV infections, the typical infected American woman is likely to experience one of these incurable STDs as a severe stress on her sense of wellbeing. This negative shift can occur even at the receipt of a diagnostic result, which merely indicates the possibility of HPV infection: Zimet (2006, 23) documented "the emotional suffering associated with abnormal Papanicolaou (Pap) test results." In a U.S. society, which supports a double-standard of sexual behavior and, consequently, a sexist magnification of the negative impact of STDs for women, a clinically minor problem (like an abnormal Pap result) can quickly become a cause for major concern.

Most Americans subscribe to a gender ideology in which girls and women are morally and socially demeaned by non-marital sexual encounters, whereas these same behaviors serve to elevate the social statuses of boys and men (Eyre, Davis, and Peacock 2001). Sexual health researchers find that the traits which U.S. society associates with contracting STDs—"indiscriminate promiscuity, pollution, and uncleanness" (Lawless, Kippax, and Crawford 1996, 1371)—are incongruous with cultural definitions of feminine 'goodness.' In this climate, a woman with a lifelong STD tends to become fearful about how others will view her.

Chronic STDs as Turning Points in Women's Lives

To understand how women view themselves with chronic STDs, I use the theoretical lens of *symbolic interactionism* in which, "Identities are meanings attributed to self, by others and by self. They are developed in interaction as others respond to particular presentations of self" (Kelly 1992, 395). An *interactionist* would say that how we see ourselves and how others see us are interdependent concepts because we construct personal identities through social interactions. Contracting an incurable sexually transmitted disease creates a "turning-point moment" (Strauss 1959) for most American women, in that the illness initiates an "identity dilemma." As Charmaz (1994) found, "Identity

dilemmas result from losing valued attributes, physical functions, social roles, and personal pursuits through illness and their corresponding valued identities" (269). In many social contexts and social roles, a
person's sexual health status may have little, if any, impact on how they
view themselves or how others view them, but STDs present a particular threat to an individual's *sexual self.*

Damaged Goods draws on women's firsthand experiences to explore how social constructions of female sexual morality merge with
stereotypes about STDs to threaten women's *sexual selves*: Individuals'
views of themselves as sexual beings that exist in relation to their general views of themselves. My conceptualization of a *sexual self* draws
on components of Dowd's (1996) theory of a *secret self*: "Privacy allows
individuals to have a secret self, which may be a sphere of behavior
that is engaged in behind closed doors, out-of-view, and which the actor would prefer to keep separate from the public sphere" (249). In this
sense, the term "sexual self" signifies a typically private self, shaped by
emotions, cognitions, and memories of sexual experiences.

I conceive of the sexual self as encompassing individuals' self-
evaluations of their own sexual desirability and how they think of their
own imagined and experienced erotic sensuality. Other researchers
have posited similar operational definitions of the term *sexual self*
(Breakwell and Millward 1997; Cranson and Caron 1998; Sandstrom
1996) to refer to something fundamentally different from a gender
identity or a sexual identity. I agree with Breakwell and Millward that,
"the structure of the sexual self-concept is significantly influenced by
dominant social representations of gender differences and relationships" (1997, 29).

While a few other researchers and theorists have referred to the
sexual self-concept, this term's definition has not been agreed on. I
posit the components of a sexual self to include the level of sexual ex-
perimentation, emotional memories of sexual pleasure (or lack thereof),
perception of one's body as desirable or undesirable, and perception of
one's sexual body parts as healthy or unhealthy. Research has yet to
explore why the sexual self is uniquely susceptible to damage. Applying
Goffman's (1963) concept of a "spoiled identity," I propose that STDs,
in addition to other traumatic experiences, may create, add to, or
maintain a *spoiled sexual self*, resulting in both intrapersonal and interpersonal costs: these traumas include molestation, rape, homophobia,

self-loathing brought on by social constructions of attractiveness, and other sexually-related medical conditions (e.g., infertility, breast cancer, and impotency). Social interactions that communicate that some physical bodies are less attractive, particular sexual preferences are unacceptable, or certain levels of sexual experience are immoral, can also transmit messages that damage sexual selves. *Damaged Goods* expands on the work of medical sociologists (Charmaz 1994; Sandstrom 1996; Swanson and Chenitz 1993) by examining how these women are transformed during each stage in their illness experiences. At each of the six stages, particular factors create, maintain, challenge, and reshape how they see themselves as sexual beings.

The Roots of STD Stigma

Ancient Greeks used the descriptive term "stigmata" to refer to visible marks which signified the bearer as one who was tainted and deserved to be ostracized. Manzo (2004) clarified Goffman's (1963) conceptualization of stigma by looking for the qualities that made social scientists likely to label a condition as "stigmatizing." He determined that STDs fit the criteria of being stigmatizing because of contagiousness and culpability. Manzo highlights a key point of Goffman's earlier work, "that stigma attaches not only to persons but to specific social contexts" (Manzo 2004, 414). Stigma is not simply a discrediting attribute; rather, each stigma is the product of a process of social interactions within a cultural context.

Centuries before the first case of HIV/AIDS, the social stigma and health ramifications of other sexually transmitted diseases scarred the lives of many around the world. The experiences of U.S. women and men today must be seen in historical context. Sexual health services in the U.S. became strongly influenced by moral objectives when, in the late1800s, male physicians "professionalized" midwifery. The growing preference and respect for scientifically educated male professionals in the field of women's health allowed for sexist moral agendas to shape American medical philosophy and public health services related to STDs. Public opinion and public health campaigns have often targeted sexually active, working-class and minority women as the "vectors and vessels" of sexual disease (Davidson 1994; Luker 1998; Mahood 1990). Scholars have elaborated on the class dynamics of these campaigns. For example, Ehrenreich and English (1973) found that Victorian-era upper-class women received an abundance of medical care, whereas lower-class women received almost no general health care services. However, the lower-classes, and lower-class *women* in particular, have been viewed as the transmitters of disease to the wealthier classes.

During the social hygiene movement of the Progressive Era (1890–1913), physicians and women moral reformers combined forces to explicitly shape the moral boundaries of sexual behavior, under the justification of public good/health. However active the women reformers may have been, these boundaries were decidedly sexist. The doctrine of "physical necessity" was deemed to justify, and often excuse, men's forays into promiscuity. As early as 1910, Dock pointed out the bias in how the (then popular) *theory of innate depravity* was applied to "fallen women" and not to their male counterparts, whose sexual escapades were equally, if not more, shameful than those of the women.

Historical documents reveal that, during this period of the early 20th century, physicians had constructed a spectrum of culpability, positing "innocent patients" at one end—those children and married women who had been infected via an adulterous husband—and infected married men and "problem girls" at the other end (Davidson 1994). Not only had these "problem girls" contracted diseases willfully, but they were also the "major vectors of disease" by virtue of their promiscuity and low morals.

This view of women regained momentum in the 1980s when early AIDS research studies viewed women "not as victims of the disease but as risk factors to others," and the public regarded HIV infections in women as "simply the natural consequence of the way they choose to live, the 'wages of sin'" (Nechas and Foley 1994, 98; 101). A recent overview of findings from qualitative studies of HIV-positive women asserts that women's experiences of HIV-related stigma were intensified because they were female: They had been socialized to believe in gender norms and values that meant that their social relations and moral identity were threatened by others' awareness of their infection status (Sandelowski, Lambe and Barroso 2005). Beyond HIV, studies have examined the gendered nature of American attitudes toward other STDs, looking at the interplay between negative social constructions of

STDs and culturally defined gender roles in differentially shaping patients' experiences of diagnoses, symptoms, and treatment (e.g. Meyer-Weitz et al.1998). Eng and Butler (1997) have argued that sexual mores *explicitly* shaped public health policy and are reflected in past and present societal attitudes toward sexual health. Society's focus on assigning moral culpability to illness encouraged policy makers to ignore the social and environmental factors that contributed to disease and reinforced the tendency to reject, ridicule or simply ignore those who suffer from an illness.

A few researchers have charted social histories of the moralization of STDs (Brandt 1987; Davidson 1994; Luker 1998) and illuminated issues of social power and subordination. Others have examined the ways in which public perceptions of health policy and practice have reflected social acceptance of the sexual subordination of women (Lock and Kaufert 1998; Lorber 1993). The social history of sexually transmitted diseases in the United States reflects a tradition of not only assigning moral responsibility to those infected with STDs, but also of differentially assigning moral stigma on the basis of gender, race, and class (Brandt 1987; Luker 1998).

Social stereotypes of sexual immorality and disease are specific to sex, gender, ethnicity, and socioeconomic status. Researchers have found that biased norms of sexual morality have influenced a wide range of sexual health programs: "Current campaigns against STDs which are aimed at women are infused with the same moral judgments found in earlier campaigns" (Leonardo and Chrisler 1992, 1). In addition to inaccurately targeting populations for outreach, biased health research has increased the likelihood that the more complex issues faced by individuals with STDs will not be addressed. For example, Lock (2000) explained how the targeting of certain populations on the basis of ascribed traits, such as sex and ethnicity, sets the stage for medically ineffective and socially destructive health policies and programs. She cautioned that it becomes easy to overlook true inequalities, like poverty, when we are comfortable blaming individuals' biological traits, such as ethnicity and sex, for their designation as 'high-risk' groups for particular diseases.

Thus we need to examine women's experiences of STD diagnostic and treatment interactions within a larger social context (including race/ethnicity, socioeconomic status, religious identity, age, etc.) of how female sexuality and sexual morality have been constructed in the United States. In line with Mechanic's (1989) conceptualization of illness experiences as "shaped by socio-cultural and social-psychological factors," my research explores women's experiences of chronic STDs within medico-moral interactions that are shaped by race, class, and gender norms of sexual health and behavior.

Sex, Gender and STD Stigma

Feminist scholars have highlighted the resilience and salience of gender: "despite the impact of feminism and deconstruction, gender has not been abolished, but continues to be reinscribed in our identities, desires, and thought" (Thomson and Holland 1997:2). While it is true that gender norms may be influenced by norms of race/ethnicity, sexuality, age, etc., a woman negotiates her sense of self and identity by referring to and measuring herself against the gender norms that have been constructed as most important in her life experiences. Hughes (1945) conceptualized a "master status" as a social identity that is dominant and influences the way in which individuals are viewed. As long as being a woman is one's master status in common contexts (e.g., intimate relationships, the gynecologist's office, and motherhood), then one is expected to meet stereotypical expectations of femininity, including sexual behavior norms and sexual morality norms.

Looking back at the late 19th and early 20th centuries, the meaning of 'femininity' created categories for women on either side of the sexual morality dichotomy: "God's police" posed in opposition to "damned whores" (Summers 1975). Historically, these labels gave one group of women a sense of duty to keep a critical eye on their *sinful* sisters and to dole out stigmatizing labels when necessary. Current debates about surveillance and sexual health question the value of public health professionals labeling certain groups as 'at-risk'(O'Byrne and Holmes 2005). This type of labeling has been linked to promoting sexism, racism, and homophobia, both inside and outside the U.S.

Researchers on AIDS in Africa found significant gender differences with regard to stigma: "Popular ideas about STDs suggest little stigma is attached to male infection. Having an STD is almost regarded as a rite of passage into manhood, proof of sexual activity: 'A bull is not a bull without his scars'" (Bassett and Mhloyi 1991, 143). These researchers found that African women experienced greater degrees of stigmatization and ostracism as a result of a HIV infection. Other researchers, looking at the gendered implications of non-HIV sexual transmitted diseases, confirmed that, "women feel particularly shamed and isolated as a result of the infection" (Pitts et al. 1995, 1303). A recent study of adolescents' views of sex found one ideology to dominant among young women and young men: "the gender ideology linked with the 'double standard' in which males are morally elevated by multiple sexual encounters, while females are morally demeaned" (Eyre, Davis and Peacock 2001, 13).

Across cultures, sexually transmitted diseases have been connected to promiscuity. The traits our society has traditionally associated with contracting an STD—promiscuity, irresponsibility, uncleanness, immorality, and even naïveté—were incongruous with cultural definitions of being a "good" girl/woman. In this way, the context of gender is especially important for understanding both the social construction of sexual disease in the United States and why contracting a STD, especially an incurable one, can be a severely stigmatizing illness experience for women.

Goffman (1963) discussed stigma as contextual phenomena: "Not all undesirable traits are at issue, but only those which are incongruous with our stereotype of what a given type of individual should be" (3). From a symbolic interactionist perspective, individuals intersubjectively create meanings about STD infection during interactions. For example, interactions between medical practitioners and lay people have been found to be the conduits through which STD stigma are reinforced (Brandt 1987). Social constructionist, labeling and conflict theories enhance our understanding of how people come to understand different illnesses: individuals and social control agents (e.g., medical practitioners), "construct particular acts as deviance and individuals as deviants" via processes that entail the creation of and sharing of meanings (Best 2006). *Damaged Goods* illuminates important facets of stigma in the "moral careers" (Goffman 1959) of female STD patients.

Social prejudices have been found to intensify against individuals, such as those infected with STDs, who were believed to have caused their own stigmatization (Goffman 1963). Tewksbury and McGaughey

(1997) applied this concept to the development of HIV-related stigma. They contended that the physiological and social qualities of this disease make it likely for persons living with HIV to experience the three faces of stigma as put forth by Goffman (1963, 4): "Abominations of the body . . . blemishes of individual character . . . tribal stigma." Given the global devastation resulting from HIV/AIDS, the majority of contemporary scholarship on chronic illness, moral identity, and the self has focused on this disease. However, *Damaged Goods* is the first book to focus exclusively on the social-psychological impact of two other incurable STDs. While the physiological impacts of these viral infections differ greatly from HIV, I argue that genital herpes and HPV infections similarly challenge women's perceptions of themselves with regard to health, morality, and social status.

Medical Sociological Studies of Sexual Health

American sexual health policies and attitudes have always been shaped, in part, by prevailing medical beliefs and practices. In the 1970s, American cultural views of health shifted from a focus on germ theory—that certain microorganisms cause disease—to an emphasis on individual responsibility for behaviors that might cause disease. Epidemiological studies from that period show that behavioral choices, such as smoking and exercise, influence ill health. "No longer would disease be viewed as a random event; it would now be viewed as a failure of individual control, a lack of self-discipline, an intrinsic moral failing" (Brandt 1997, 64). The ways in which both medical and lay people speak about particular diagnoses have often denoted blame and individual responsibility to the sick. When we feel comfortable blaming the sick for their own illnesses—if their own 'bad' choices caused their health problems—then the rest of us who are making 'good' choices can all feel less at-risk.

Along with scholars who have documented the popularity of blaming individuals for their own poor health, researchers have also examined the role of medical practitioners in the social construction of health and illness. Medical practitioners, for example, in addition to controlling health information and services, also have the capacity to serve as social control agents, in that they have implicit authority to assign moral statuses to different illnesses. Early work on hospital staff documented the prevalence of "moral evaluations" of patients (Roth 1972). Foucault (1978) argued that social control in the field of medicine had become more professionalized and oriented to the surveillance of deviant behavior. Social responses to STDs illustrate how medico-moral discourses have served to construct and regulate sexuality (Foucault 1978, Mort 1987, Davenport-Hines 1991, Davidson 1994).

Pryce (1998) pointed to a critical gap—the "missing" sociology of sexual disease–and asserted that this application of sociology should focus on the social construction of the body as central in the medical and social understandings of STDs. Sociological research on sexual morality and health has primarily addressed HIV/AIDS (Fernando 1993; Matthews 1988; Nechas and Foley 1994; Plumridge and Chetwynd 1998; Ray 1989). The overwhelming focus of social scientific studies of STDs, other than HIV, has been on evaluating the effectiveness of education/prevention strategies, environmental determinants, and understanding risk assessment and risk-taking behaviors (e.g., Beadnell et al. 2006; Rogers 1999; Shrier et al. 1999; Thomas et al. 1999).

Most research on morality in the socio-medical politics of STDs has addressed the issue from a national level. Few studies examine micro-level interactions in sexual health services, especially from patients' perspectives. Such studies can illuminate issues that occur at the interface between medical practitioners and patients. As such, qualitative studies have not fully examined affected individuals' "illness behaviors," which Mechanic (1982) defines as "the manner[s] in which persons monitor their bodies, define and interpret their symptoms, take remedial actions, and utilize the health-care system" (1). A more recent study focused on how the stigma of sexually transmitted diseases may affect one particular illness behavior—that of seeking treatment for STD infections. Lichtenstein (2003) found that African-Americans' willingness to access sexual health treatment at public health facilities was directly and indirectly impacted by STD-related stigma: specifically, religious ideation, privacy fears, racial attitudes, and the fear of being "scarlet lettered" proved to impact individuals' willingness to seek medical treatment.

The practitioner-patient interactions that comprise STD diagnoses differ from other chronic illness in that there are explicit and implicit threats of negative health *and* negative moral consequences. A study on media coverage of herpes in the early 1980s found that the stories stressed "a psychological and social deadliness"—evidence that the detrimental effects of herpes diagnoses extended beyond the physical (Signorielli 1993, 60). Medical research determined "the most common and usually the most devastating problem of having genital herpes is its psychological impact" (Bettoli 1982, 925). However, most studies of individuals infected with herpes have neglected to address the identity impacts of the physical, moral, and social consequences of receiving a diagnosis (Reiser 1986; Rosenthal et al. 1995; Swanson and Chenitz 1993). Two recent articles (Melville et al. 2003; Breitkopf 2004) confirmed the presence and ramifications of stigma experienced by individuals living with genital herpes. The later concluded that the stigma experienced by those living with herpes will lessen as we see more media portrayals of these individuals as normal and the infection as treatable. For example, recent commercials for *Valtrex*, a popular antiviral medication, have portrayed infected individuals as active (e.g., riding mountain bikes) and happily involved in intimate relationships (e.g., embracing a significant other while professing their understanding that even correct and consistent use of this medication does not guarantee protection for an uninfected partner).

With regard to HPV, most studies of affected individuals focus on risk evaluation/risk-taking behavior (e.g., Ford and Moscicki 1995). One clinical study (Keller et al. 1995) advised practitioners to be aware of the psychosocial aspects of HPV diagnoses, but did not examine why these negative implications exist or how they might affect patients in different ways. While this study noted the "potentially traumatic nature of HPV infection" (Keller et al. 1995, 356), my study is the first to fully analyze the social-psychological impacts of having HPV. A more recent study noted that HPV-related stigma may create feelings of embarrassment and fear of rejection, which could lead to infected individuals choosing not to disclose their HPV-positive status to sexual partners (Keller et al. 2000). This dangerous public health consequence of STD stigma emphasizes the urgency for a more complete understanding of how being diagnosed with a chronic sexually transmitted disease may affect the self-concepts and decision-making processes of infected individuals.

For the past two decades, interactionist medical sociologists have studied first-hand accounts of illness experiences. Analyses of chronic illness, in particular, have led to the creations of theories about the social and psychological consequences for those affected. Several scholars have examined the challenges posed by chronic illness to self and identity (e.g. Charmaz 1994; Frank 1991; Sandstrom 1996). Medical sociologists have specifically explored the impact of stigma by focusing on how chronically ill individuals manage both identity dilemmas and interpersonal relationships (Conrad and Schneider 1980; Tewksbury and McGaughey 1997; Weitz 1991).

Interactionist studies of chronic illness have begun to explore sexual-self concepts. For example, Sandstrom (1996) sought to fill an important gap in the literature on the self in chronic illness by exploring how HIV/AIDS, "affects the sexuality and sexual identity work of diagnosed individuals" by examining men's "sexual self-images" (242). Other research on HIV/AIDS has looked at how the diagnosis serves to redefine not only affected individuals' health statuses, but also their sexual statuses (Sandstrom 1990; Weitz 1991). These scholars have documented redefinitions of self and status; however, none of these researchers have addressed infections, like genital herpes and genital HPV, which are lifelong but manageable. *Damaged Goods* details the different ways in which these sexually contagious and highly stigmatizing infections transform women's sexual selves.

Genital HPV and herpes infections, as sexually stigmatizing chronic illnesses, pose specific challenges to infected women's selves and identities. Pioneers in researching the connection between self-conception and sexual health, Swanson and Chenitz (1993) used qualitative methods to examine the relationship between herpes infections and a "valued" self, which began analysis at the point of diagnosis. While these researchers theorized a three-stage model of regaining a valued sense of self after herpes diagnoses, their findings indicate a more complex process that begins well before the point of contracting an STD and is shaped by social dynamics of gender, race, class, sexuality, etc. In *Damaged Goods*, I aim to detail six stages of how chronic STDs transform women's sexual selves and include stages prior to diagnosis.

On Methodology: Researching an Invisible Population

Motivated by personal experience, I entered this research setting as a "complete member" (Adler and Adler 1987). At age 20, I was diagnosed with a cervical HPV infection. In fact, the prose "snapshot" that began this chapter is actually the beginning of my own story.[10] Self-education helped me to manage the initial stress of diagnosis and treatment. Then, volunteer involvement with sexual health education and outreach became the foundation for my research and provided me with insights and legitimacy to connect with others facing STD diagnoses. Ultimately, I worked as a professional a sexual health educator, and I drew on these experiences for the clinical knowledge necessary to understand and interpret the women's illness narratives. (See Appendix A for a complete discussion of my auto-ethnography.)

As a professional sexual health educator in the late 1990s, I began to question how individuals infected with chronic STDs managed the intrapersonal and interpersonal challenges. To more fully understand the social and psychological impact of chronic STDs on women, I aimed to uncover how these women created, maintained, and transformed the meanings of their STD illness experiences. My goal was to collect data that could provide an empirical foundation from which to test the prevailing medical, sociological, and lay assumptions about women living with chronic STDs.

Women with STDs are a hidden population, their identities protected by medical confidentiality. Aware of the negative social attitudes toward infected women, most keep their sexual health statuses a secret. In this sense, their stigmatized condition is *discreditable* (Goffman 1963), and the women can *pass* as sexually healthy in most social contexts. With this norm of secrecy, women with non-HIV STDs are also a fragmented population, unlikely to engage in support groups or identity politics for fear of outing themselves.

Having conducted a survey study that found women strongly preferred maintaining the confidentiality of their sexual health statuses, I determined that one-on-one interviews were the best method of data collection. As this topic is sensitive and laden with sociocultural "baggage," talking with these women individually created an intimate research space in which I had the best chance for high construct validity. In this manner, I was able to develop what Blumer (1973, 798) described as, "a close, flexible and reflective examination" of contemporary social facts about women with STDs. The data I collected can be conceptualized both as *sexual stories* (Plummer 1995) and as *illness narratives* (Frank 1993), in that each woman spoke about intimate, sexual, and sensual aspects of her life; while she also described her encounters with the medical profession as a patient being treated for one or more STDs.

As with many studies of individuals living with HIV/AIDS (e.g., Cranson and Caron 1998; Grove, Kelly, and Liu 1997; Sandstrom 1996), I employed a mixture of convenience and snowball sampling (Biernacki and Waldork 1981) because of the research topic's sensitive nature. In keeping with the principles of grounded theory, I sampled for theory construction, rather than for representativeness (Charmaz 1995). In all, I interviewed forty-three women who had been diagnosed with genital herpes and/or HPV infections for this study. My final sample size resulted from ethical restrictions on subject recruitment: I was not allowed to actively recruit subject; rather I could only post flyers, print ads, and announce my study when giving public presentations on sexual health. Given doctor-patient confidentiality, there was no way for me to obtain a list of the women who met the sampling criteria and then engage in any form of random or purposive sampling. In sum, due to the sensitive topic, medical policies, and research ethics, I was limited in my ability to create a more diverse sample.

The women who participated in my study ranged in age from 19 to 56 years old at the time of their interviews. Though these participants comprised a convenience sample, my goal was to interview women who varied in how they identified with regard to ethnicity, socioeconomic status, religion, and sexuality. I viewed these categories of characteristics as being highly relevant to the exploration of meanings for feminine sexual morality and sexual disease, in addition to potentially impacting the women's experiences of and options for sexual health care. In terms of ethnicity, thirty-eight identified as European American (including Jewish, Greek, and Persian ethnicities), three as Latinas, one as African-American, and one as Native-American. Socioeconomically, they ranged from upper-class (1) to working class (9), with the majority identifying as lower-middle (5), middle (18), or upper-middle (10) class.

The participants represented a variety of religious upbringings and current practices: Buddhists, Jews, Muslims, Pagans, and Christians (Catholics, Protestants, and Southern Baptists). Catholics (12) were the largest group, but fourteen women had been raised with no religion, and nineteen reported being currently nonreligious. With regard to sexual identity, the majority (37) identified as heterosexual, five identified as bisexual, and one identified as a lesbian. (See Appendix C for more detailed information about the participants and research methodology.)

In-depth, semi-structured interviews allowed me the flexibility in the data gathering process to uncover what having a chronic STD meant to this sample of women. Constant comparative analysis (Glaser and Strauss 1967; Glaser 1978) provided the guidelines by which I was able to ferret out the shared meanings of STD stereotypes, symptoms, diagnoses, and treatments from the subjective point of view of those living with these infections and accompanying social stigma. Utilizing a symbolic interactionist approach to guide my data collection and analysis, I tested emerging hypotheses about the empirical realities of women with STDs, via a thorough and continuous examination of their world (Blumer 1969).

While their identities are protected by pseudonyms in this work, the details of their stories are exactly as they told them to me. No story is identical to another, but many shared similar motivations for participation in this research: (1) To help others by giving voice to the real struggles of millions of women who live with these infections, and (2) To personally benefit from managing their STD stigma, via cathartic disclosure, relief from the burden of secrecy (Adler and Adler 2006). My goal, in sharing their stories, via sociological analysis, is to frame their individual struggles within a larger, social context and highlight opportunities for improvement in sexual health education and medical services for women and their sexual partners. (See Appendix B for a detailed methodology discussion.)

Organization of the Chapters: Six Stages of Sexual Self-Transformation

Damaged Goods draws on in-depth interviews with women who have been diagnosed with genital HSV and/or HPV infections. Highlighting the voices of these women, I write about the transformations of their *sexual selves*—how they see themselves as sexual beings—and how they understood and made choices about sexual health issues. I document the physical, moral, and social consequences of living with these diseases, by analyzing their experiences within a six-stage framework. I use symbolic interactionist, social psychological, and feminist theories to explore the ways in which these women's sexual-selves are transformed throughout their STD illness experiences.

In Chapters 2 through 7, I draw on the women's stories to illustrate the six stages of sexual self transformation. Each of these chapters explains a different stage in how the women constructed STDs as meaningful in shaping their sexual selves and interpersonal relationships. The women I interviewed came from a variety of backgrounds, but common threads emerged, as illustrated by their quotes and anecdotes, that conveyed the interplay between socio-demographic factors, cultural constructions of health, gender, and sexual morality, and structural norms of the American medical system.

I created a model that illuminates stages in the "moral careers" (Goffman 1959) of STD patients and documents the event series that ultimately shape changes in patients' sexual selves and social relationships. This theoretical model represents "ideal types" in the sense that not all women went through each stage in the same manner, and the following chapters detail and analyze variation between individuals' experiences. In stage one, *Sexual Invincibility*, early portions of women's socio-sexual histories create and maintain beliefs in a myth of STD immunity. In stage two, *STD Anxiety*, women's experiences of initial symptoms or practitioners' suggestions of possible infection replace feelings of invincibility with anxiety. In stage three, *Immoral Patient*, they experience practitioners' deliveries of STD diagnoses as imparting health, moral, and social stigma. In stage four, *Damaged Goods*, women employ individual stigma management strategies within interpersonal relationships. In stage five, *Sexual Healing*, they face the interpersonal, physical, emotional, and financial challenges of treatments. Finally in stage six, *Reintegration*, many women reconcile the meanings of their illness experiences by integrating risk awareness and desire for intimacy within revised sexual selves.

Damaged Goods expands discussions of moral identity and sexuality in chronic illness by examining genital herpes and HPV from social-psychological and interactionist perspectives. Highlighting the role of social power, it focuses on how their illness experiences serve to create "turning-point moments" (Strauss 1959) in the women's narratives of their sexual selves. By interweaving their stories, via sociological analysis, *Damaged Goods* creates a virtual community for women who have felt alone in their struggles for health, self-acceptance, and sexual intimacy. Ultimately, I hope that this work contributes to a widespread de-stigmatization of these illnesses.

2 Sexual Invincibility

aving interviewed women from a range of backgrounds (age, class, race/ethnicity, etc.), I expected a substantial amount of variety in their descriptions of early memories of learning about sex and sexual health. However, similar means, methods, and messages pertaining to sex education and socialization emerged from the data. All of the women recalled feeling they were invincible when it came to sexual health prior to the point in their lives when they contracted their first STD.

The women's shared false conceptions of STD immunity can be linked to American values and norms of female sexuality. Noting women's feelings of invincibility toward HIV/AIDS, Chrisler and Leonardo (1992, 6) hypothesized a societal cause:

> To see AIDS as a threat to herself, a woman has to accept the fact that she is sexually active. This may be particularly difficult for young women in a society that has traditionally divided good women and sexual women into different groups. Women who are taught to feel ashamed of their sexuality may also be likely to deny it.

My research showed that this causal dynamic is at play in understanding U.S. women's perceptions of general STD risk. The stories of the women I interviewed were interwoven with societal expectations, stereotypes, and distinctions that led them to want to see themselves as "good" girls who should not have to worry about the shameful health problems of being sexual and, therefore, a "bad" girl.

To chart out the stage of *sexual invincibility*, the first stage in my model of sexual self transformation, I analyzed several components of the women's early life histories. First, I explored how the women came to learn the meanings of female sexual behavior and risk, via formal and informal interactions. Their institutional, cultural, and interpersonal experiences combined to create a myth of STD immunity. Next, I examined the women's descriptions of childhood and adolescent sexual experiences that provided evidence of how the myth was maintained or refined without disrupting beliefs in STD immunity. Finally, I synthesized the dangerous consequences of such a myth: Their sexual attitudes and behaviors based on feelings of invincibility set the stage for why these women contracted STDs and the stressful process of how STD illness experiences would transform their sexual selves.

Creating the Myth

All of the women were raised and educated in the United States. Their attitudes and beliefs about sex and health were shaped both by formal institutions, such as schools and churches, and by interpersonal relationships with parents, siblings, and peers. In this section, I examine the women's answers to my question: "How did you first learn about sex and sexual health?" Their answers reflect variations in generational attitudes toward sexuality, diversity in private and public educational backgrounds, and differences in parental ideological outlooks (very conservative to extremely liberal).

Formal Sexual Health Education

In her examination of the politics of sex education, Thomson (1994) argues: "Sex education is potentially a vehicle for social engineering par excellence, be it progressive or traditional" (40). She highlighted the power of formal institutions in creating the foundations of sexual attitudes and behaviors. The women I interviewed reported a wide range of sex education experiences: From none at all, to focusing solely on puberty, to discussing contraception and STDs.

The data reflected historical changes in American sex education policies: Women who graduated high school after 1980 reported having participated in more comprehensive sex education programs, women who graduated high school prior to 1980 represented most of the cases of absent or limited sex education. However, a few of the women under 25 years of age reported having had little or no sex education by virtue of having grown up in rural areas or having gone to Catholic schools.

Approximately 25 percent of the women reported having received no formal sex education through twelfth grade. Pam, a 42-year-old, white, working-class graduate student, grew up in the late 60s and said she did not receive any sex education in her public schools. As Lily, a 40-year-old, white, middle-class graduate student and mother, put it, "In my generation, I'm forty, sexual health wasn't something we were taught." She reflected on the cultural expectations of young women in her generation:

> So it's just alarming me because I'm still not sure I have all the information I should have, and I'm a pretty well-informed person. So that really concerns me for the whole generation of women my age 'cause we were never taught . . . it was something that you just kind of didn't talk about back in the 50s . . . and if you ask questions like that of doctors, you would have been considered a bad girl. And, of course, I went to the family doctor that knew my family. I wasn't gonna ask those kind of questions!

Similarly, Gloria, a 47-year-old Chicana graduate student and mother, did not have any formal sex education but looked to her peers for information, or misinformation as the case may have been. "We had what we heard from each other . . . lots of stories." All of the other women described a range of educational content and quantity, with some having received sex education in elementary school, and others having had their first formal curriculum in high school.

Elementary School

Sex education during elementary school years most often consisted of a film focusing on puberty, emphasizing different changes for boys versus girls, with the boys and girls separated for the viewing of these films. As Marissa, a 31-year-old, Hispanic, lower-middle-class graduate student, described it: "The girls went off and saw a little film, it's from about 1950 or something, you know, about your period. And, basically that was about it." Many of the women remembered being shown this sort of video as early as the fourth grade. Some of the women also received class instruction ranging from basic to in-depth knowledge.

However, Violet, a 35-year-old, white, upper-middle-class engineer, did not even get to see the standard film. "In sixth grade, [my teacher] told us about how all girls were going to get wide hips like hers. And, we were all going to get periods, and she showed us a chart with fallopian tubes and stuff. And, that was about the extent of it." Slightly more informed, Ingrid, a 23-year-old, white, middle-class undergraduate, remembered her "first true sex ed class" being in the fifth grade. "That was not addressing STDs or anything. That was merely addressing sort of girl parts versus boy parts, menstruation, wet dreams and stuff, that sort of really biological thing."

In contrast, Haley, a 22-year-old, white, upper-middle-class undergraduate, had a week of fifth grade devoted to "sex ed" where the education was a bit more in depth:

> They split up all the girls and all the boys . . . and she had some movies. She had some little pamphlets and handouts, brought in the box of pads and the box of tampons and a box of condoms . . . but she barely touched on like birth control and things like that. It was mostly like how the female and male reproductive systems work and what happens when this thing called "a period" comes.

Haley described her peers' reactions that reveal the meanings 9- and 10-year-olds derive from these educational programs:

> We all just thought it was kinda' funny. Yeah, it was like pass around the tampons and stuff. It was kind of the big joke,

and then afterwards we'd all get back in the hallway and girls met up with the boys and there'd be all kinds of jokes and comments flying around the hallways about pads and erections.

A challenge of elementary school sex education lay, not only in the limited content, but also in the maturity level of the audience. However, Haley and others who received puberty-focused sexual health education in elementary school reported feeling well prepared for the arrival of menstruation.

Middle School/Junior High School

The women who received sex education in middle school/junior high recalled more of a focus on pregnancy prevention, but STDs remained relatively invisible. Anne, a 28-year-old, white, lower-middle-class graduate student, remembered a health class in junior high that was focused, "around pregnancy and reproductive functioning, but I don't remember much information about sexually transmitted diseases." However, a few of the women had more breadth in their sex education. Following the initial education described in the preceding section, Haley also had a multi-week course in seventh grade that spanned several controversial issues of health. "The focus was birth control and STDs, like HIV and the whole sharing-needle thing. It was kind of drug education as well." However, when I asked her how meaningful this information felt to her seventh grade self, she said, "It seemed so distant." At this point, she did not personally know anyone who had gotten pregnant or contracted an STD. "It was kind of strange material in a way. . . . All these crazy things can happen to you. . . . But, yeah, it seemed so distant that it almost went in one ear and out the other."

Sexual health educators employed a variety of techniques to make STDs feel more tangible. One example was using slide shows and/or photos of genitalia that were severely infected with STDs. Robin, a 21-year-old, white, upper-middle-class undergraduate, went to an all-girl school and remembered guest speakers coming with slides and pictures of genitals with "pieces falling off" because the individuals had not taken care of their infections. While she contended that these educators "brought everything . . . diaphragms and jellies . . . everything so you could see it and play with it," she admitted that they did not show condoms or demonstrate the proper use: "They were not allowed to bring a dildo." Her case illustrated how school district policies can potentially decrease their effectiveness by limiting content of programs. Catholic schools presented a special case of limited sex education programming. Francine, a 43-year-old, white, middle-class health educator, remembered her limited education in junior high school:

> I didn't even have a good picture of what having sex was about. Because, in a Catholic school, the boys were separated from the girls, and the only information we got had to do with having your period . . . the only thing I'd gotten was the eighth grade booklet about your menstrual cycle.

Diana, a 45-year-old, African American, upper-middle-class professional, shared recollections that paralleled Francine's in pointing to an underlying philosophy that knowledge about sex would lead to adolescents having sex:

> All I remember from Catholic school was that you weren't supposed to do it, you know. It was kinda' like keep your panties up and don't even think about it. To think about it might have even been a mortal sin, you know what I mean? . . . It was certainly all this stuff about it was a sin and you shouldn't even be thinking about that.

The women who attended Catholic schools consistently described explicit lessons about the link between sexual behavior and morality.

Ingrid, while a generation younger than Diana and Francine, recalled her first STD educator, a nun, as having had a similar perspective:

> I think that I knew it was a fairly good education, but so much of it was presented like, "You don't have to worry about it because you won't get it anyways because you're a good Catholic." . . . I remember AIDS was the only STD discussed: pregnancy and AIDS pretty much. I mean AIDS was a big

deal. But it was also, from the perspective of the teachers, "Well, you're a good Catholic, so you won't get it."

In addition to connecting sexual behavior with morality, these examples suggest that Catholic schools engendered a belief in STD immunity by virtue of differentiating between different types of people: those who "sinned" and therefore had to worry about pregnancy and STDs, versus "good" Catholics who did not have to be concerned.

Race became a factor in Ingrid's sex education when her school invited in a guest speaker from a local AIDS organization focused exclusively on AIDS impact on "people of color." This presenter "showed slide after slide, photographs of various infections on various parts of the body . . . a baby who had been born with gonorrhea . . . warts and herpes." While she recalled how she and her classmates had been "affected by it for weeks," she remembered discussions with her peers about believing that once they were married, STDs would be a non-issue. In addition, Ingrid recalled how racial stereotypes became connected to sexual disease by virtue of this slide show presentation.

> A bad thing about the presentation was that most of the photographs were of people of color . . . and it's probably sort of subconscious, but if you see a bunch of warts on a Black man's penis . . . I think that has a big factor . . . I know that probably there is a higher risk of STDs in communities with less money, and I supposed you can link communities of less money to people of colored skin . . . I know, in that class, that's probably the first, last and only time that most of those people will ever see the genitals of a Black person or Mexican.

Due to the guest speaker having highlighted STDs as a problem that affects people of color, Ingrid, as a white student, feared that the other white students would see people of color as diseased and in turn, not see themselves at risk.

The age at which moral meanings became attached to STDs was fairly consistent among the women. While a few recalled overhearing other's comments about STDs prior to sixth grade, all cited middle school (or junior high school) as the time when their sexual health ideologies took shape. When asked what ideas they had then about sexually diseased people, their descriptions matched a primary myth found in Cline's (2006) study: "STDs, including HIV, only happen to people who do bad things or make bad choices" (354).

High School

Those women who received sexual health education in high school often learned more about STDs, in addition to contraception. However, the content and quality of this education varied greatly depending upon the era and the social values of the school district. Very few of the women who were over forty had any high school sex education. Diana switched to a public high school after going to Catholic schools since kindergarten. In public high school, she learned about syphilis and gonorrhea in high school health class, but also saw herself as immune:

> I knew that they were there. But I didn't ever think that, I would be around anybody who would have anything like that . . . just kind of scum people had it. You know, and men who hung out with prostitutes. Just like your regular, everyday guy shouldn't have syphilis or gonorrhea.

Middle school and high school teachers, either through explicit lessons, or via the absence of certain information, had the power to educate their students about STDs, such that they learned to view these diseases as *other people's problems*. In the large majority of cases, the result was a removal of this health problem from the students' perceived realities.

Those who had received high school sex education before the mid 1980s, prior to HIV/AIDS becoming a topic of public school education, described a similar content of curriculum. Caprice, a 35-year-old, white, clerical worker, graduated high school in 1981 and remembered "herpes was the big deal," a sentiment expressed by many women who were in high school during the end of the "Disco Era" when herpes exploded as a national epidemic. She had graduated high school in 1983, before HIV/AIDS was nationally recognized as a health problem. Cleo a thirty-one-year-old, white, middle-class graduate student and mother, remembered that her health class featured "this little film on VD [venereal disease]" that discussed gonorrhea and syphilis, but ignored HPV/genital warts and herpes. This fact was particularly disturbing because the medical community had already recognized these two diseases as serious epidemics at the time (Brandt 1987; Keller et al. 1995). Elle, a 32-year-old, white, working-class graduate student, had also graduated high school in 1983 and described having seen a similar film: "The big [STDs] at that time were gonorrhea and syphilis [portrayed] like Disney cartoons: the little gonorrhea and syphilis germs putting on helmets and going to war inside the body." Similarly, Tasha, a 30 year-old, white, middle-class graduate student who graduated high school in 1984, learned about syphilis as a disease which meant "people going crazy" and about gonorrhea as a curable infection. However, her teacher "definitely drummed home the condom thing" and reinforced her perception that "STDs are avoidable as long as you use condoms."[1] She linked this early lesson on condoms as one of the main reasons she did not perceive herself as at risk for contracting an STD before she was diagnosed.

The women I interviewed who graduated high school after 1989 described a wider range of content in their high school sex education. Jasmine, a 20-year-old, white, upper-class undergraduate, had seen guest speakers from Planned Parenthood who created an open atmosphere in which she and her classmates could have their questions answered:

My freshman year, they had two volunteers from Planned Parenthood come in and talk to us. And they were actually two girls that we knew from our school, and they were talking about various aspects of sex. It was really neat to hear somebody being that open with it . . . to see that people weren't embarrassed about [sex], they could talk about [sex] and educate other people.

However, at this point in time, she was planning to "save" herself for marriage. Due to this sexual self-conception, Jasmine felt that the guest speakers' messages did not reach her.

I didn't really think it applied to me, but I thought it was really neat they were sharing their stories because I knew that, at that point in time, some of my more distant friends had had sex, and we had talked a little bit about it. But, still, none of my closest friends had [had sex].

Sex and all of its dangers were not a part of her intimate surroundings. Gita, a 23-year-old, Persian American, middle-class administrative assistant, similarly felt that the guest speaker who "came in and talked about contraception and safe sex" to her sophomore class did not seem relevant to her. In contrast, Sandy, a 21-year-old, white, middle-class undergraduate, learned "about anatomy, they taught about STDs, how to put a condom on, and abstinence." She definitely felt concerned about pregnancy because she had become sexually active in eighth grade. However, like Tasha, Sandy learned that "[she]couldn't get an STD if [she] used a condom."

While the women I interviewed are older than today's typical undergraduate student, a recent study has found that current sex education trends in the U.S. reflect a return to the sex education content that was more typical in the 1970s and 1980s. Federal funding and policies promoting abstinence-only sex education have had a significant impact in recent years. Researchers at the Guttmacher Institute compared survey results on adolescents' sexual education experiences from the years 1995 and 2002: Rates of adolescent females receiving formal education about birth control fell from 87 percent to 70 percent, and the rate of those receiving abstinence-only education rose from 8 percent to 21 percent (Lindberg, Sing, and Finer 2005). So, these women's stories likely mirror the current range of experiences for adolescent females today.

Informal Sexual Health Education

Schools were not the only venue for sexual health education experiences. As Monica, a 21-year-old white middle-class undergraduate, stated, school taught her "none of the sex stuff: That, I would say, I learned from social relationships rather than institutions." Just as important, if not more important, STD lessons came from the women's childhood interactions with parents and peers.

Parents

Not all parents were open to talking with their daughters about sex. In these cases, the women learned what was right and wrong both from what their parents said and did not say. Francine, who had gone to Catholic schools, remembered that while her mother would often tell her, "If you have questions, come to me," she did not feel comfortable seeking her mother out for answers about sex. She saw her parents as "going along with what they thought was the way to go, which was, 'Just don't give them any information that they don't need because if you give them information they may become interested in sex.'" Silence about sexual health prevailed in many of the women's childhood homes, even when it came to matters of menstruation. Gloria, a Chicana, working-class, single mother, had also been raised Catholic, and said that her mother was not only unwilling to discuss sex, but she gave minimal guidance to help her daughter understand her first period.

> When I started my period, I had to knock at the door and tell my mother I was bleeding. And my mother said, "Go open the closet, the blue box with some white pads in there. Get one of those pads on you. Go in the bathroom and put it in your underwear." And I said okay, but I thought I was bleeding to death. So I didn't understand what was happening . . . I just figured okay, she must know what's going on, even though I don't know.

The absence of sexual health education at the family level helped to render sex a mystery, leaving these women more open to believing what their peers had to say about pubertal changes, pregnancy, and STDs.

Some socially conservative parents found ways to talk with their daughters and reinforce traditional values and morals. Amelia, a 26--year-old, white, middle-class graduate student, shared her memory of being an eight-year-old and a talk with her mother: "I remember my mom talking to me about the whole kind of clinical birds and bees thing . . . And, I remember her specifically saying sex was something that happened within the context of marriage." Other less conservative parents found it easier to rely on books to bridge the communication gap with their daughters. For example, Summer, a 20-year-old, lower-middle-class, Native American, remembered coming home from a class on menstruation at 11 years old:

> My mother was sitting in a recliner in the family room, and she had books stacked up to the top of the armrest on both sides. And she says, "Come here. We need to talk." . . . And she explained to me, even more in depth than school was allowed

to, what happens when a man and a woman have sex. That the man ejaculates, and she gave me the whole facts of life story from every book in the library she could find.

One advantage to this technique is that it taught the women that sexual health education could be found in a library or bookstore; this approach to seeking sexual knowledge would help them later on to clarify and dismantle misinformation about their own STDs.

Some parents were "forced" to teach their daughters about sex by virtue of unplanned learning opportunities. For instance, Diana's mother, who was a conservative Catholic and had "always been a little uncomfortable talking about sex,"found herself having to explain sexual intercourse to a five-year-old Diana:

> I was at the park, and some couple was having sex in the daytime. And, the blanket blew off of them, and I saw the man with this *thing*. So I went home and told my mother and she was trying to chill me out 'cause I was totally like, "What was that?" . . . She did calm me down. She gave me some explanations.

Similarly, Sam, a 34-year-old, white, working-class graduate student infected with HPV, remembered that her mother had explained sex to her when she was in the second grade. The catalyst for their talk had come from a young Sam needing help on the writing of a story about "how baby horses were made."

Other parents and grandparents taught their daughters explicitly about the connection between sex and morality. Janine, a 50-year-old, white, middle-class graduate student, had been raised as a child by her grandmother. "You were supposed to be a virgin when you got married and that was very important to them. As I got older, it just didn't seem very important at all [to me], and they did definitely make chastising comments about my sexual choices. It wasn't fun." For Haley, only four years out of high school, the memories of sexual condemnation by her father were still fresh. He had falsely accused his daughter of "losing [her] virginity and having sex all the time." His accusations began in ninth grade when Haley admittedly began having problems "getting along" with her parents. In a misogynistic manner, her father took out his frustration with her by saying things like, "I think you're a little whore." She remembered the pain of his targeted accusations: "When he said to me, things like that, it just cut you know. It hurt the worst." These sexual lessons were gendered, outlining the expectations for *good girls* and punishments for *bad girls*.

A few of the women described interacting with parents who were more liberal and open-minded about sex. Rebecca, a 56-year-old, white, upper-middle-class professional, attributed her parents openness to the fact that they were "very rational and scientific, or tried very hard to be, in their approach to everything, and I was encouraged to read for myself—anything I wanted to." This policy extended to sexuality when a young Rebecca came home talking about a book that her girlfriend had not been allowed to read. "They checked out what the book was and decided to buy it for me, and it was a very, very sanitary, very cute little book called *Growing Up*." Her parents made it clear that they would be happy to buy her additional books and discuss the issues. For different reasons, Lola, a 30-year-old, white, lower-middle-class sales person, remembered feeling very comfortable asking her mother questions about sex and attributed her mother's attitude to cultural differences.

> I think I became sexually aware and educated at a much earlier age than most people in this country. I'm gonna' stereotype here because my mom was European, and they have very different attitudes about sex. I mean she caught me lots of times masturbating, messing around with my girlfriends, and playing doctor . . . and she never made me feel bad about myself. She just kinda' let me do it because she knew that it was a natural growing part of the curiosity and discovery of your body.

Overall, the data reveal that women experienced more open sexual education experiences with parents who had higher levels of education and were from more permissive cultural and/or religious upbringings.

Peers
For all of the women, friends and other peers provided sounding boards, sources of knowledge, and safe havens for questions about sexual health. As Kelly, a 31-year-old, white, middle-class graduate

student, stated, "Sex wasn't talked about in our family . . . so, if anything with sex comes up, it was, pretty much, conversations between me and my best friend." Peers were sources of both accurate and inaccurate sexual health information, playing key roles in shaping the women's youthful perceptions of sexual invincibility.

For some of the women, all health risks were absent from their memories of sexual talk with their junior high school and high school peers. Gloria, who had grown up in a strict Latino Catholic family, asserted, "We didn't even hear about STDs. We never knew what they even were." Kelly, whose alcoholic father and neglectful mother set few boundaries, covertly watched pornographic movies with her best girlfriend as an adolescent but did not remember STDs being part of the fantasy world they observed. Summer had a military father who was often overseas and a working mother who usually got home late, so she lacked parental supervision. She became sexually active at age 13 and only remembers her girlfriends pressuring her to have sex by telling her, "You've got to try it. You're gonna' love sex. We know once you start having sex, you're gonna' love it." None of these friends cautioned her about pregnancy or any health risks.

Other women recalled minor references to sexual health risks, with more of an emphasis on pregnancy. Deborah, a 32-year-old, white, upper-middle-class counselor explained that when she was 13, she "vaguely remember[ed] hearing you could get bad things from sex." When asked for clarification, she explained that she knew pregnancy was one "bad" outcome but was unsure of others. Diana talked about how, in the early 70s, her high school friends talked "about guys and, you know, they had these *things* that could make you pregnant." She had no memories of STDs coming up in these discussions.

However, some of the women had friends who talked explicitly about the health risks of sex. Elle learned about STDs and the benefits of condoms from a junior high rumor about a girl "who was sleeping with the boys in seventh grade and had diseases, but the boys knew if they were gonna' sleep with her to just put on a condom, then they wouldn't get the disease." She conceptualized STD prevention based on the 'moral' of this story: "You can sleep with a *skank*, just make sure you protect yourself." Rhonda, a 23-year-old, Cuban American clerical worker, had high school friends who taught her a similarly incomplete lesson when they told her to, "use condoms and be safe," if she had sex.

She "didn't know specific things, like what terms go with what and what's not treatable," so she, like Elle, did not know that condoms still left the risks of herpes and HPV transmission.

A few of the women talked about friends who discussed STDs with them in more detail because they were infected. For example, Ingrid "had a couple of gay friends" in high school who, in addition to telling her and her girlfriend how to "give better [oral sex]," talked about HPV because one of them had contracted it from a sexual partner. The openness about sexuality speaks to the looser sexual norms of the 1990s. She also had a girlfriend who contracted herpes at 16 and another who contracted HIV at 19. While these experiences made STDs seems like a real part of their peers' lives, the women differentiated themselves from these friends and how they conducted their sex lives. Illustrating this differentiation, Ingrid believed that only people who had sex "with an unreasonable amount of people" were at risk. Her sexual plan was to "wait until [I am] twenty years old and totally in love because having sex with one person is not gonna' get you an STD." Ironically, she would go on to later contract HPV from her very first love, her first sexual partner, after "saving" her virginity until she was 20.

The Resulting Myth

Lessons learned in school, from parents, and from peers taught the women about sex, but did not add up to produce an accurate picture of sexual health risks. All of these sources left the women feeling afraid of some aspects of sexuality and excited about others. In general, the resulting foundation of sexual knowledge with which the women left high school contained more danger messages about pregnancy than STDs.

Vulnerability to Pregnancy ... Not to STDs

For many of the women, the focus on contraception came from knowing young people who had dealt with unintended pregnancies. Gloria, 47 years old at the time of our interview, remembered how her parents, peers, and others in her Mexican-American neighborhood would gossip about how "so-and-so got pregnant from so-and-so . . . and what a horrible thing it was." As a result, she "always feared being pregnant."

Monica explained that pregnancy "seemed real" in her middle-class, white, suburban neighborhood because she "knew this girl that had two abortions within four years of high school." Caprice described the class bias growing up in a wealthier neighborhood: STDs "only happen to people of the city or people who sleep with ten million people, and it wouldn't happen to anyone I know because we're all upper-middleclass." This compartmentalization of sexual risk by social class left her feeling afraid of accidental pregnancy, but not fearing STDs. "I just never knew anyone who had a disease, so it didn't seem very real. Whereas you heard about some people getting pregnant, so that was real. I needed an example in order to believe it."

Parents also reinforced the focus on pregnancy, seeing their daughters as vulnerable in that regard. For 34-year-old Sam, "pregnancy was definitely a fear" when she was first becoming sexually active in high school. However, she felt comfortable talking with her liberal mother who told her, "If you're gonna' become sexually active . . . make sure that you're using some kind of birth control." Sam's mother never cautioned her to be wary of STDs. On the opposite end of the parental spectrum, Diana's strict Catholic parents added the threat of punishment to solidify her fear of pregnancy. "I was scared. I felt like my father would kill me if he found out." She also connected unintended pregnancy with preventing her from attaining her education goals. "You know, I wanted to get away . . . wanted to go to college, and I felt like if I started fooling around with [my high school boyfriend], I was really gonna' be in trouble." While the thought of pregnancy conjured up fears of losing educational opportunities, she had no fears of contracting an STD. "You know, STDs weren't that big of a deal [in the 1970s]." According to the women who graduated high school in the 80s and 90s, their later generations also did not worry about STDs, other than HIV/AIDS.

The Role of HIV/AIDS Education

Several of the women who graduated high school in the late 70s to early 80s commented on how pregnancy was emphasized over STDs, in both formal and informal sex education experiences. Deborah reflected on how her few sex education classes had "drilled into our heads that you could get pregnant from one time sex." Lola attributed this bias in her education to having graduated high school just as AIDS arrived on the public health agenda:

> I don't think STDs even became an issue until towards the end of high school . . . the primary thing that people were worried about was pregnancy. And, my senior year in high school was when the AIDS epidemic began, and I really think that it was the manifestation of AIDS that kind of brought in the whole awareness of STDs in general because before that, I can't say that I ever even heard of [herpes].

When I asked her if she knew of any friends who had been infected with an STD, she replied, "No, no. It was always pregnancy."

However, the women I interviewed who graduated high school well after the beginning of the U.S. HIV/AIDS epidemic did not report a significant shift in education about other STDs. Natasha, a 20--year-old, white, middle-class undergraduate, remembered "people talking about certain people that got pregnant," but did hear "one rumor that flashed by" about someone having AIDS. "Other than that, I don't remember any STDs being talked about or people having them. Just that people got pregnant or that someone had an abortion." As opposed to Natasha's informal AIDS education, Ingrid, who graduated high school in 1995, remembers learning about AIDS as part of her Catholic school's sexual health curriculum and viewing this disease as something that she could contract:

> I saw myself at risk for AIDS and only for one reason: because they always say, "It can happen to you." But I never thought herpes. I mean interestingly enough, HPV being such an epidemic, it was easily the one I worried least about . . . I think the reason why I never liked to think of myself as susceptible to such things, and probably most people don't, is that [educators] never addressed what you did once you had it. It made it sound like if you got herpes, no one was ever going to have sex with you. No one was ever going to love you or find you attractive.

She drew on this gap in STD education to explain that she never thought she was going to "get it" or had to "watch out" because people with STDs would not be mistaken for sexually desirable. In addition, the repetition of HIV/AIDS awareness campaign messages that "anyone can get this disease" made an impression on Ingrid and other women of her generation that this was the only STD worth worrying about. Once the women evaluated themselves as not participating in one of the "top" risk behaviors (IV drug use, sex with bisexual men, etc.) their feelings of invincibility were renewed.

Maintaining the Myth

Sexual innocence is a precarious state during childhood and adolescence. Both consensual and nonconsensual sexual experiences test and shape individual's attitudes about sex and sexual health. The women recounted sexual experiences from their youth that reinforced, transformed, or destroyed their feelings of general sexual invincibility. However, the data reveal how these women gave meaning to both pleasurable and traumatic experiences, such that their feelings of STD immunity remained untouched.

Sexual Innocence: Reinforcing the Myth

Approximately one-third of the women described their sexual development and experiences through high school as consisting of consensual and enjoyable activities. The women in this subgroup remembered awakening to their sexuality as a gradual progression, marked by steady transitions. For example, Lola recalled feeling "frisky" as a young girl and viewed her awakening feelings in a positive light:

> I always had crushes on people . . . I had this huge, huge crush on my cousin and then when we came to the United States, I had this huge crush on my other cousin. And, then, when I started watching TV, there were always certain people that I was just infatuated with.

Her early "crushes" were experiences where she felt in control of desiring another because she was safe from any interaction actually occurring.

Not being sexually victimized as children or adolescents allowed these women to engage in the normative transitions of sexual expression at each stage in their development. Janine compared the 1950s sexual norms and expectations of her peers in elementary school versus middle school:

> I remember kissing boys in first grade on the playground . . . it certainly wasn't particularly sexual at that point. But around sixth grade, we started having little boyfriends and held hands and stuff, and then you realized, beyond that the bar got raised. You had that little spin the bottle party and stuff like that.

Rhonda, who attended elementary school in the 1980s, similarly conceptualized this time in her life: "Fifth and sixth grade for me were really sweet years." She remembered being clear with herself that "there was no desire to do anything, not even to kiss." She felt comfortable being true to her desires and maintaining comfortable boundaries.

A few of the women talked about how they had engaged in masturbation and consensual sex play with other children their age. Lola and a girlfriend "played a lot of doctor with each other" before they were nine years old. They even went so far as to explore orgasms, which they called "good feeling":

> This whole thing with good feeling was we'd sneak off into the camper . . . and, we'd crawl up in there, and we would totally mess around and get naked and touch each other. And, say things like "How does that feel?" and just be messing around like that.

Elle related that her first sexual memory was of masturbating at the age of four. She was "caught" by her mother who chastised, "That's dirty." However, she found a quick remedy that, to her mind at the time, dealt with her mother's concerns and allowed her to continue experiencing pleasure: "I washed my hands afterwards." As both of these women exemplify, parental and societal messages that discouraged children from seeking out sexual pleasure did not stop their quests, rather they adapted their behaviors to evade detection. The power to be sexual and enjoy their sexuality remained theirs. As they entered adulthood, positive childhood experiences further reinforced their beliefs that nothing "bad" would happen to them in the sexual realm.

Sexual Victimization: Refining the Myth

Approximately two-thirds of the women disclosed memories of childhood and/or adolescent sexual trauma as having tested, altered, or destroyed their feelings of general sexual invincibility. However, while these experiences damaged their feelings of sexual power and safety, their feelings of STD immunity remained untouched.

Even seemingly minor traumas, such as sexual harassment, left indelible stains on the women's beliefs about their personal power and ability to protect themselves. Natasha remembered several incidents in middle school when she was "sexually harassed on a bus." The boys had originally targeted another girl who was "of the lower-class" and "had big boobs." Feeling at this point that her class status and lesser-developed body made her immune to their attacks, Natasha was shocked when they switched their venomous attention to her: "I was kind of shy, and they wanted to get under my skin." Their attacks included asking her "is your pussy stretched?" She took this as a blatant accusation about her chastity but felt trapped by her feminine role of wanting "to please and be liked." Likewise, Amelia, whose mother had explained sex to her when she was eight years old, cited gender norms as the reason why she tolerated "being blatantly sexually harassed" by boys. She felt uncomfortable being "grabbed" and "fondled," but wanted "attention" from boys and wanted a boyfriend. She "felt guilt" over wanting this attention and thought of herself as a slut for allowing the harassment to continue. Diana illustrated a racial dimension of being sexually harassed:

> I had some bad experiences with white men as an adolescent, particularly down south where I was approached by white men asking me to have sex for money . . . I think it turned me off of white men in general to think that somebody would come up to me and offer me money for sex just because I was a Black woman.

She learned that white privilege magnified male sexual privilege. As a woman of color, she was automatically more vulnerable than a white woman.

Approximately 10 percent of the women told stories of attempted rape, successfully fighting off both strangers and acquaintances. However, over half of the women in my sample were raped, molested, or victimized by incest. At age nine, Diana was molested by a sixteen-year-old neighborhood boy, but remembered enjoying the positive attention that came from "sitting on men's laps." Her parents found out and were angry with Diana: "My parents really got on my case . . . I always sort of felt like I was the one being punished, in part, for that." From this experience, she learned that, even if she were the victim, she could face negative consequences in the form of condemnation for having been tainted by sexual immorality. Kelly was also molested in the fourth grade and "felt ashamed" because she and her girlfriend "kept going back" because "it felt good" to have male attention. Again, the gendered nature of sexual roles set girls up to crave male attention, even if it meant being molested. Even the women who experienced date rape as older teenagers expressed feeling similarly torn. Caprice was raped at nineteen by a man who wanted to take her virginity. She recalled, "the spooky thing about that was I still wanted to be around him even after that 'cause I figured it was about time [to lose my virginity] anyway." Caught on the double-edged sword of feminine sexual morality, facing ridicule for being either a prude or a slut, Caprice was partially relieved to have gained sexual experience, even at the cost of her feelings of sexual control and power.

The consequences of enduring sexual trauma, as either a girl or young woman, included a range of intrapersonal and interpersonal consequences. Pam had been molested by a teenaged boy in the neighborhood when she was 5 years old. Until she was 30, she was "very guarded" around teenaged boys and men. She attributed this feeling scared to her associated sexual attention with their being predators. Anne's first sexual experience was losing her virginity at 12 to a 17-year-old boy. Too young to have truly given consent, she admitted that she "felt pretty violated and certainly developed a really negative image of sex at that point." She left this experience believing that sex was "painful and if you go a little bit into it, that means you're ready to go all the way." Both of these women illustrate the powerlessness that comes from surviving sexual assault.

Other survivors of sexual assault expressed feelings of *disassociation* during later consensual sexual encounters. After being date-raped as a teenager, Natasha tended to emotionally and cognitively withdraw whenever she tried to be sexual. "It made me develop a pattern where I began to withdraw in my mind, you know, while I was performing my sexual acts or while I was being intimate with someone." She tended to enter this state of mind when "things got a little bit too rough, where I didn't want to be there." Violet, a 35-year-old, white, upper-middle-class engineer, had been a victim of incest committed by her father from age three; she describes using a similar coping mechanism when she later engaged in consensual sex: "I just checked out . . . We were having sex, but I didn't have any feelings in my body . . . my body was just way too scared . . . I was just emotionally disconnected."

Surprisingly, as these experiences of sexual trauma and assault made this subgroup of women feel vulnerable, with regard to their sexual power and safety, they nevertheless continued to feel invincible with regard to STDs. Their stories highlight the power of formal and informal sexual health education: With STDs absent or minimally present in their early lessons about sex, the myth remained untouched, even when other aspects of their sexual self-concept were damaged.

Consequences of the Myth

Growing up with consistent messages that consensual sex is safe so long as you protect against pregnancy, and experiencing no interactions that cast doubt upon the veracity of the information they had received, the women entered adulthood feeling that they were immune to STDs. In turn, this belief translated into feeling and ultimately acting as if they were invincible in this regard. Their actions included sexual behaviors that put them at high risk for contracting genital herpes and HPV.

Feeling Invincible

The women expressed a variety of justifications that explain their feelings of sexual invincibility. Their feelings of immunity derived from incorrect medical information, stereotypes of individuals who contract

STDs, age-related generalizations about prevalence and risk, being "in denial," and surviving curable STDs without long-term consequences.

While both the herpes virus and human papillomavirus spread, via skin-to-skin contact that can occur without penetrative intercourse, many of the women reported feeling safe from all STDs, so long as they did not "go all the way." Robin explained that, because her sexual health educators had stressed penile-vaginal intercourse as the only way in which one could contract a disease, she believed STDs only "happened to other people . . . because I hadn't been doing anything . . . I hadn't had intercourse so I'll be fine." Ingrid similarly expressed, "basically when I left that high school classroom, my thought was that if you did not have sex, you could not get an STD." Because her educators "never addressed what you did once you had [an STD], it made it sound like if you got herpes, no one was ever going to have sex with you. No one was ever going to love you or find you attractive." She extrapolated from what her educators included and excluded, and she remarked that her conclusion that STD-infected people did not have sex was "the reason why I never even thought of myself as susceptible." If infected individuals were celibate, then how would she ever end up having sex with an infected person?

Another dimension of invincibility came from how the women saw themselves in relation to the stereotype of the type of person who contracts and spreads STDs. Jasmine, 20-year-old, white undergraduate, reflected on the socioeconomic norms of her upper-class community. "I thought, coming from where I did, that it was only dirty girls or sluts that would get [STDs], and I definitely never thought that I would end up with it." Ingrid paralleled this idea of class-related immunity when she admitted that she left high school believing that STDs only infected those at "the bottom of the barrel." Elle, who lost her virginity at age 20, mirrored this sentiment: "Well, I didn't think of myself as a *skank*, and only *skanks* got STDs. So, apparently, I wasn't going to get an STD because I was protected by the *unskankiness* shield. Nice girls didn't get it."

Age also played a factor in engendering invincibility. A few of the women who graduated high school in the 80s remembered graduating and feeling that STDs were diseases solely transmitted among older people. Helena, a 31-year-old, Greek-American, middle-class graduate student, noted, "The only things we knew about were like syphilis and gonorrhea, and that was kind of what older people got." On the opposite end of the spectrum, a few of the women who graduated high school in the 60s credited their feelings of immunity to being from an older generation. Rebecca thought that STDs happened to people, "who were younger, who were still courting around much more than I was." Because of this belief, she "didn't have any particularly negative attitudes towards sleeping with a variety of people" so long as she knew the person she "was sleeping with and had at least some feelings for them."

A few of the women acknowledged that denial played a role in their feelings about STD vulnerability. For example, Natasha, who had been sexually harassed as a teenager, admitted that she had come to view herself as "one of those girls that was sleeping with a pretty good amount of people," so she could have easily seen herself as fitting the STD stereotype of promiscuity. Instead, she "tried to avoid the thought of STDs . . . I denied the issue so it wasn't about who was a person that could have an STD. I was very invincible." Similarly, Amelia remembered that she first learned the term *slut* in association with girls who "slept around" and likely had STDs. However, even when her peers later labeled her a slut, she still did not see herself at risk.

At an extreme level of denial, that demonstrates the strength of the myth of STD immunity, almost half of the women contracted one or more curable STDs prior to contracting herpes or HPV. However, even these first-hand experiences with the reality of risk did not change their attitudes. For example, Violet contracted a bacterial STD while in traveling in Germany, but did not change her attitudes because antibiotics effectively cured it. Caprice contracted Chlamydia but felt that, since it was curable, "it was a fluke." Their belief in sexual invincibility remained intact.

Acting Invincible

As the women entered adult sex lives from a firm foundation of invincibility, feelings of STD immunity translated into sexually risky behaviors. Never having been formally taught or informally socialized to place themselves in the category of "people at risk," almost all of the women interacted with sexual partners as if STDs were not a possibility.

Many of the women described practicing unprotected sex—sexual intercourse without proper and consistent use of latex condoms. Violet described the time in her life when she was 18–21 years old: "During that period, I had a lot of sexual partners, and I totally felt like I was invincible. I didn't take any precautions whatsoever." She attributes her behaviors directly to her foundation of sex education and socialization, having come of age "a while back, before STDs were a big deal." When Helena had her first sexual experience at fifteen without condoms, she remembered "a positive feeling . . . I don't think I ever thought of being intimate with someone as a bad thing." Chris, a 40-year-old, white, middle-class professional, remembered having a lot of partners in her early 20s: "[Sex] was positive, freedom at that time . . . it would be very common to walk into a room or a bar and have slept with most of the men there." She was consistent with contraception but did not protect herself against STDs.

Several of the women connected their risky sexual behaviors to having learned inaccurate information about STDs. Amelia recounted an experience of deciding to have unprotected intercourse with a male partner even when she knew his last partner had genital warts. She described her mindset at the time: "I didn't know that her warts were a virus. Like she had them lasered [sic] off, and I knew they never came back, so I never even thought about [contracting HPV]." Tanya, a 27-year-old, white, upper-middle-class graduate student, recalled trying to be cautious about sexual health with her boyfriend by asking if he had been tested for STDs. He replied, "Yes, all of it." However, even though "he said he had been tested for everything, what he was tested for, I'm not quite sure." No educator, parent, or peer had ever told her which diseases could be detected by readily available tests: Most clinics cannot definitively test for genital herpes or HPV when the virus is latent (asymptomatic).

Reliance on stereotypes about STD-infected people also provided rationalizations for engaging in unprotected intercourse with partners that were presumed to be "clean." Natasha elaborated on why she felt she knew how to pick safe partners: "Sometimes it depended on who the guy was . . . this really nice guy, I liked him, I trusted him, so he should know what his standing is," with regard to STDs. In these cases, she felt safe relying only on birth control pills for contraception. Similarly, Jenny, an 18-year-old, white, upper-middle-class undergraduate, was only concerned about getting pregnant by her high school boyfriend until she found out he had cheated on her, "with a girl who we all knew was promiscuous." I think one of my first thoughts was about STDs because I didn't think she was a very clean person . . . she'd had sex with so many people." Before Jenny became aware of his infidelity, she had thought she would never have to worry about STDs, so long as she dated boys from "good" families. In a different but equally effective manner, the six women who had had sexual relationships with female partners, used stereotypes that lesbians were "STD-free," to justify the absence of latex protection during sex. Anne, who identified as bisexual, joked that since there were no concerns about birth control, she had no need to talk about sexual health issues with her female partners.

Learning the myth of sexual invincibility from trusted authority figures and valued friends, the women felt secure in basing their sexual attitudes and behaviors on this false foundation of STD immunity. Experiencing sexually "innocent" childhoods only served to reinforce this myth. At the same time, sexually traumatic childhoods spotlighted many of the pitfalls and dangers of sex but left the issue of sexual disease in the shadows. Entering adulthood with the assumptions detailed in this chapter, the women went forward in their sex lives with no reason to doubt their core belief in STD invincibility, until troubling symptoms or unexpected news gave them a reason to worry.

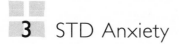

3 STD Anxiety

aving lived with the idea that STDs only infected "other" types of people, the women all had clear memories of abrupt transitions: From feelings of invincibility to feelings of anxiety about sexual health. They entered the stage of *STD Anxiety* when they first became alerted to possibilities that they may have contracted genital herpes or HPV. The women described how the presence or absence of symptoms shaped their emotional reactions to the possibilities of STD infections: From denial to acceptance and urgency. They also discussed betrayal as an interactional variable that increased the negative emotional impact of this pre-diagnostic stage. Contextual elements created frameworks of discovery, within which the women experienced differing levels of pre-diagnostic anxiety over their dawning medical realities.

Absence or Presence of Symptoms

For some of the women, outward symptoms (genital warts and/or herpes lesions) signaled to them that their bodies had been possibly infected. However, many of the women, who would eventually receive HPV diagnoses, reported having experienced no noticeable symptoms at this pre-diagnostic stage and were surprised to have their sexual health called into question.

Asymptomatic Infections

HPV infections are often asymptomatic with the ability to remain latent for several years after initial contraction of the virus. For this reason, approximately half of the women in the study, all of whom would later receive HPV diagnoses, had no idea they had been exposed to, let alone contracted, a chronic STD. Their bodies displayed no noticeable symptoms.

A few of the asymptomatic women were alerted to the potential of having contracted HPV through interactions with their past or present sexual partners. Marissa, a Hispanic graduate student, discussed how, years earlier as an undergraduate, she had received a call from her ex-boyfriend who said, "I was watching 20/20, and they had this thing on about warts . . . well, you know, I noticed something on my penis, and it sounds like what they're talking about on the show." This conversation triggered the beginning of an anxious time, wondering whether or not she had been exposed to and contracted genital warts. However, Marissa felt fairly certain that he had not contracted HPV from her: "My first reaction was, well, I don't think it was from me. And I was asking him about other people that he had dated, you know, 'cause he wasn't real big on using condoms.'" Marissa and other women in similar situations would have to wait for a medical practitioner to confirm their STD status before knowing whether or not they had definite reasons to worry.

In contrast, the majority of the women in this subgroup were surprised by medical practitioners' suggestions that they had STD infections. Within contexts of annual gynecological exams, they sought routine Pap smears, totally unaware that they had been exposed to, let alone contracted, a chronic STD. Since social class is part of the myth—that poor and working-class women are more likely to be infected—some middle—and upper-class women noted that their practitioners had never previously advised them to seek out STD testing. "The false assumptions about who is at risk for HIV/STD infections affect screening and counseling practices of public and private healthcare providers. While STD and HIV screening and counseling are a regular part of the standard of care in local public health departments and community health centers, it is normally not a part of routine screening in many private practices" (Cline 2006, 354).

Approximately half of the women in this subgroup recalled low levels of anxiety resulting from practitioners' pre-diagnostic hypotheses that they had likely contracted cervical HPV. For example, Molly, a 43-year-old, white, middle-class undergraduate, admitted that she "didn't know that much about [Pap smears]" at the time, when she received her first abnormal Pap smear result. She rationalized that she had been "having Pap smears for a reason" and "figured this [possibility of abnormal cells] is why you have a Pap smear." Personally, Molly knew that she and her husband had both been virgins when they married and had been faithful during their marriage. Her one possible cause for STD anxiety, a rape that occurred a few years into her marriage and several years prior to this exam, felt so distant that she did not believe her Pap smear result could be anything related to an STD.

The other 50 percent of the women, who had been asymptomatic prior to being alerted to a possible STD during their annual exams, recalled feeling high levels of anxiety over news of an abnormal Pap smear result. After Jasmine's second abnormal Pap smear result in a four-month time period she was "really scared." Then she read a magazine article about cervical cancer and its link to HPV, and thought "Oh, my god! I can't believe this is happening to me!" Only 20 years old, her fear felt real because her aunt had had cervical cancer, and she knew about "the possibility of having to have a hysterectomy." Cleo, whose high school sex education had n ot addressed HPV, also experienced high levels of pre-diagnostic STD anxiety. She had never had a Pap smear, and went in at age 19 for her first gynecological exam, in order to get a diaphragm for birth control. A couple of months after the exam, an unusually long delay, she found out the results:

> They did the Pap smear and it came back abnormal . . . this is my first Pap smear, so I was like, "Abnormal? What does that mean?" They were using all these words: dysplasia and condyloma. And, of course, I didn't know what any of them were.

The nurse delivered these pre-diagnostic hypotheses over the phone, and Cleo felt "really scared, like I was sure it meant something awful." In her confusion over the medical jargon, she thought she had cancer. Too shocked to ask for clarification during this phone call, her confusion would not be cleared up until she returned for her diagnostic appointment.

Cleo clarified that the delay in receiving the exam results heightened her pre-diagnostic anxiety. She had been promised that Pap smear results would reach her in a matter of weeks, not months, and worried that the passage of months had increased her likelihood of her condition having progressed. Louise, a 28-year-old, white, middle-class graduate student, also received delayed notification of an abnormal Pap smear when a nurse called to tell her that her most recent "Pap smear didn't come back okay" and that her previous one, six months earlier, had also shown evidence of abnormal cervical cells. Louise panicked at this abrupt news that she had been mislead to feel sexually healthy, "and then all of a sudden" her practitioner made it sound urgent to schedule a follow-up visit to confirm a diagnosis.

In a more extreme case of practitioner negligence, Lola, 30 years old at the time of the interview, received a "very alarming letter" from her gynecologist that said:

> That he's following up with me about the results of my last Pap test, and that he urgently needs to speak with me because—he didn't say what was wrong. He just basically alluded to the fact that it's about your Pap smear, and something is wrong with you that needs to be taken care of immediately and to call me.

Lola "freaked out" and "dropped the letter after I read it—my heart just sank." She attributed her high level of anxiety to the fact that "this letter was to address a Pap smear that was done a year previously." She drew on her gynecological knowledge that Pap smears "are to test for cervical cancer":

> So all of a sudden it was just like—oh, shit!*** Something is wrong with me, and something has been going on with me for a year. And, it's been given that much time to get worse . . . I couldn't sleep all night. I called [my doctor] up first thing at 8:00

o'clock in the morning when his office opened and said, "Get me in now."

As the above three stories illustrate, practitioners, by how and when they informed women of STD possibilities, had the ability to shape women's emotional and intellectual meanings of their news of probable infections.

Even when practitioners acted in a prompt and compassionate manner when delivering news of a possible STD infection, the severity of the woman's condition could add to her feelings of anxiety. In a more serious case of cervical HPV, Lily, a mother at the time, had to revise her whole conception of herself as sexually healthy. "I had always been very healthy, and I've never had any, that I was aware of, known sexual disease," she commented. However, her "regular Pap smear" returned results of severe cervical dysplasia: Cervical cells radically transformed by HPV infection, such that her doctor considered her condition pre-cancerous with a high likelihood of progressing to cancer. Before she found out her condition had been caused by an STD, Lily had already gained a strong sense of the severity the situation.

While it may be easy to conceive of women not noticing cellular changes of their cervical tissue, a few of the women with external HPV (genital warts), also did not notice symptoms prior to a routine gynecological exam. As discussed in the introduction, genital warts are usually painless, close to skin color, and start off very small. Heidi, a 31-year-old, white, working-class graduate student, recalled being surprised by her gynecologist during "a routine gynecological exam" when she was 24 years old. She had made the appointment merely as a measure of health maintenance and was not prepared to hear her practitioner suggest that she had an incurable STD. When I asked her if she had noticed any symptoms, she replied, "No, none at all. And they just told me at the [clinic] that I had some external warts, and none of my Paps [sic] had come back abnormal before that time." Heidi represents the common misconception: Women often believe that Pap smears test for all genital HPV infections, and practitioners have not explained that the procedure only tests for cervical infections.

Symptomatic Infections

The remaining half of my sample noticed external symptoms prior to a sexual partner or practitioner, advising them that they might have an STD. As Mechanic (1982) noted, "Two variables define the person's estimate of the impact of symptoms: perceived seriousness and extent of disruptiveness" (15). The women's HPV and herpes infections manifested with different degrees of disruptiveness, with regard to pain and unsightliness. However, perceptions of seriousness varied, as those who experienced symptoms either reacted with denial, imagining an alternative cause for the symptoms, or with acceptance and urgency in seeking out diagnostic confirmations.

Denial

About 40 percent of the women who noticed physical manifestations of herpes or HPV tried, at first, to believe the symptoms were caused by something else. For these women, it would take official diagnostic confirmation by medical practitioners to convince them that they were infected with a virus that was both incurable and sexually transmitted. Due to less formal sex education and less exposure to media, such as, commercials, that addressed sexual health issues, the older women had grown up with less awareness of vaginal diseases (e.g., yeast infections) or STDs and were more likely to attribute their initial symptoms to transitory pain that would disappear without any medical intervention. For instance, Rebecca, who had been in a monogamous marriage at the time of her first herpes outbreak, recalled her thoughts and feelings during this time: "I was in pain, but I certainly didn't assume that it was any form of sexually transmitted disease." Janine, a 50-year-old graduate student and mother of grown children, spent the first week of her initial herpes outbreak, "trying to talk myself out of it, and then it got worse and worse." When I asked her if she knew anything about herpes at this time, she replied, "I didn't even know what this disease was . . . I knew nothing, absolutely nothing." Coming from this state of ignorance, "I figured that if I just ignored it, it was gonna' go away, and I tried not to think about it." This type of denial required an amazing amount of pain tolerance, as the longer first outbreaks of herpes go untreated, the greater the pain.

Several of the women in this subgroup attributed their symptoms to curable, non-sexually transmitted vaginal conditions when they experienced their first outbreaks of HPV or herpes. When Tanya, a "strongly Christian" graduate student, had her first outbreak of herpes, she attributed the discomfort to a yeast infection: "For the first couple of days, it was just kind of sore and itchy and I thought maybe it was a yeast infection. So I started yeast infection medication." One illustration of how meanings constructed about a first outbreak of genital warts can be shaped by interactions came from Sierra, a 23--year-old, white middle-class administrative assistant. She described how a sexual partner, directly, and gynecologist, indirectly, helped her to derive a non-STD explanation for the "bumps" she discovered on her vagina:

> I was in the shower and I was washing myself and I felt like tiny, tiny little bumps on my labia. . . . I told [my boyfriend] right away . . . and he looked at them for me because I couldn't really see them. And he's like, "[Sierra], I think it's just ingrown hairs or something. They look natural. It doesn't look like a growth." I'm like, I don't know.

In light of her boyfriend's "ingrown hairs" explanation, Sierra recalled, "I didn't go to my doctor for a few more weeks because I'd just been to her and was waiting on my Pap." She cited her doctor not having noticed the bumps at her recent appointment as further interactional proof that she did not have genital warts.

Others found more creative and unusual justifications for their STD symptoms. Julia, a 50-year-old, white, middle-class professional, lived in Thailand during her 20s and experienced her first herpes outbreak while there.

> I got an infection on my cheek. And, then, I got an infection in my eye . . . it was an open sore. And I just thought it was an infection . . . you know, there it's not uncommon to have, like, a skin infection or something like that because of the humidity and everything. I think that's what I thought it was. And I don't know if I really connected this thing with my eye thing either, but I thought they might be related.

In Julia's case, her denial of herpes was supported by her naiveté of local diseases and the unusual location of her first two outbreaks: first her cheek where an acne outbreak had left that skin vulnerable to her female partner's viral shedding, and, next, her eye which she later realized she had self-infected by touching her cheek before rubbing her eye. Julia experienced high levels of anxiety when her eye infection did not respond to antibiotic treatment and progressively worsened to the point where she thought she might lose her sight in that eye. However, it would take a doctor's diagnosis of herpes *keratitis* to connect her health anxieties to an STD. Unfortunately, during this pre-diagnostic time, she accidentally transmitted the virus from her eye to her genitals, unaware that her eye was shedding a virus that could infect her genitals.

Natasha, also, was living abroad when she had her first outbreak of genital warts and thought that she had contracted an unusual local disease.

> In Honduras, when I was showering, I discovered that I had a bump and didn't know what it was. . . . I thought maybe it was just kind of a weird pimple or something growthy [sic]. Like at first, I kind of *freaked out* and definitely thought something was wrong, but I very quickly tried to believe that it was something to do with a yeast infection. It's kind of different when you're in a third world country . . . like I have some weird disease . . . It just looked like a skin colored bump . . . it didn't itch at all.

In Natasha's case, she juggled several different justifications for why she had a wart on her labia: from natural causes (pimple), to a non-sexually transmitted disease (yeast infection), before finally rationalizing that it was a "native" disease because it did not cause her the discomfort (itching) she had learned to associate with STDs. However, in spite of all her efforts to avoid perceiving the bump as a genital wart, her emotional reaction of "freaking out" exposes the anxiety that can be present even in the face of denial.

Acceptance and Urgency
In contrast to the above interpretations, approximately 60 percent of the women who noticed symptoms of their first herpes or HPV

outbreaks reacted by accepting their sores or bumps as signs of an STD and expressed feeling urgent to get medical assistance.

Some of the women transitioned from denial to acceptance and urgency, as they confronted increasing levels of symptoms during their first outbreak. Natasha, who had originally labeled her first genital wart as first a pimple, then a yeast infection, and finally a "third-world" disease, accepted her symptoms as the signs of an STD with the arrival of an additional wart:

> Then I was in the bath one day, and I found another bump. And then I was like, "Oh, my God, oh my God, something's wrong!" The first one was still there . . . very present. [The second wart] was on the other side [of my labia]. And, so then, I started definitely freaking out. I called my mom, you know, I was upset, I was crying, and then somehow I found all these old pamphlets from high school about STDs and started looking at the ones, and I was pretty sure it wasn't herpes because it wasn't like an open like sore or anything. I had pretty much pointed it to like genital warts, but I was like also like praying that it was nothing.

As evident in her last statement, Natasha was reluctant to leave her state of denial for one of acceptance. Her emotional reaction also highlights how anxiety levels intensified for those women who reframed their symptoms as STDs.

Similarly, Tanya, who had labeled her first herpes outbreak as a yeast infection, eventually came to view it as herpes when the yeast infection treatment failed to relieve her discomfort:

> [The medication] didn't make it worse, but it didn't make it feel better . . . I didn't complete [the treatment regimen] . . . And, then I got out the mirror because it hurt to urinate and I noticed the sores . . . I thought herpes, but I'm kind of a pessimist, so I figured, I mean I don't actually know the symptoms of AIDS, but I just kinda' figured it was AIDS, too.

Tanya's case illustrated how the acceptance of the presence of one STD, herpes, can create such a high level of anxiety, that pessimism can spiral to the worst imaginable assumption even before receiving an official diagnosis of the first disease.

When Janine transitioned from trying to talk herself "out of it" to accepting that she had a serious STD, she internalized not only the medical reality of the disease, but also the moral consequences.

> The pain [got worse], and there was this moment, you know. I finally called my doctor on a Friday morning, and I was humiliated. . . . I couldn't stand it anymore . . . And, I thought, oh, my God—this is the most humiliating thing I've ever done. I actually told [my doctor] that. "I'll have to see it," that's what he said. I said, "I know I have a sexually transmitted disease."

Struck by the urgency of wanting medical assistance, Janine had to overcome not only her denial but also her pride and sense of herself as a "clean" and "good" woman as she took on the label of sexually diseased. For each of these women, the anxiety of thinking one probably has an STD quickly evolves into a premature certainty of the diagnosis yet to come.

Other women reacted to their first symptoms with immediate acceptance that they were likely facing an outbreak of herpes or HPV. Some of these women thought that they might have contracted the disease from a partner because they were suspicious of that partner's fidelity and/or sexual health status. For example, Hillary, a 22-year-old, white, middle-class undergraduate, admitted that she "definitely had suspicions" about her ex-boyfriend having "lied about everything" when she noticed a burning sensation when she urinated. She "asked to be tested for various sexually transmitted diseases" when she went in for her gynecological exam: This proved to be a wise decision because she ended up testing positive for both Chlamydia and HPV (both cervical lesions and external warts). Kayla, a 22-year-old, white, working-class undergraduate, also ended up contracting both Chlamydia and genital warts from a partner she knew had much more sexual experience than she.

> Well at the time, I was only with one partner so I know that I got both of them from him. He didn't have any like visible genital warts or anything . . . I knew something was wrong,

like this discharge, but I didn't know exactly what it was. So I went in for my annual checkup . . . and I had a couple of warts on the inside of the labia.

She had discovered the warts, via her "own detection." She explained, "Well, you could kind of see it, but it just felt weird . . . and so I was like, that can't be normal. And, I didn't think it could be anything else . . . I had heard of genital warts." These two cases exemplify how knowing the sexual experience and fidelity of a partner helped some of the women with symptoms quickly conclude that what they felt and saw were signs of an STD and promptly make a doctor's appointment.

Within contexts where one partner had been open and honest about her/his own STD status, several of the women were also able to quickly accept their initial symptoms as chronic STDs. For example, Anne, a 28-year-old, white, lower-middle-class graduate student, believed that the "tons of sores" on her vagina were in fact herpes lesions because she knew about her partner's sexual health status. In her description of how her first outbreak felt, Anne noted her partner's emotional reaction to her pain:

> It felt like my vagina was one giant sore. It was horrible! The first outbreak was really painful, *really bad.* And [my partner] felt terrible . . . it really hurt and itched a lot, and it was really uncomfortable . . . like every square inch of my vagina was covered with sores—it was awful!

Unlike Hillary and Kayla, she did not feel that her partner had been unfaithful or deceptive because he had told her about his herpes status before they had ever been sexually intimate. Due to her partner's experience and knowledge, Anne was anxious to get medical treatment and relieve her symptoms, but she was not surprised that she had contracted the virus. Francine's story also illustrates this process, as her first husband had an initial outbreak of genital warts soon after they married.

> We were in bed, and he said, "I noticed that I have this little bump here on my penis." Right on the shaft of his penis he had a couple little warts. I was clueless. I had heard about some

infections from that freshman year course, so I said, "You know, you need to go in and check this out." He probably wouldn't have gone to a doctor had it not been for me taking that course and realizing that there were some infections out there. So, he went in, and just a few days later, I ended up with warts, too.

Because she shared in her husband's experiences of STD anxiety, diagnostic confirmation and treatment, Francine "was kinda' keeping a watch out" on her own genitals and "discovered them because I was starting to get sore having sex . . . because the warts, for me, ended up being right around the opening of the vagina." She, too, was not surprised, and in fact, expected to contract the virus. Her interactions prepared her, thus she experienced low levels of anxiety during her first outbreak.

Betrayal

In addition to emotionally struggling with awakening anxieties over their transitions from sexual health to chronic sexual illness, approximately one-third of the women also had to deal with betrayal. Some found themselves in the position of being the accuser and felt deceived by an ex- or current partner. While others faced confrontations with partners who claimed they had been innocently infected.

Woman as the Accused

Not all of the women who experienced betrayal found themselves on the side of being the accuser: Several found themselves being accused by ex- and current partners of having passed on herpes or HPV. In this situation, the women's anxieties over having their first outbreaks of incurable STDs were compounded by the guilt of having infected someone else.

In Ingrid's case, she had noticed no symptoms of HPV, though she had been suspicious of her first sexual partner's penile "bumps." Rather, her current boyfriend's accusations that she had given him genital warts launched her anxieties over possibly having and passing on HPV. First, she deduced that her first partner had been the one to infect her because he "was the first person I had sex with," and she knew that her current boyfriend "was a virgin." Ingrid remembered her current boyfriend telling her:

> "I went in to get a checkup because I found something on me, a genital wart"And, he said, "I'm not accusing you of anything because I know you got tested, but I was a virgin before I had sex with you." I thought, well, my [ex-] boyfriend did sleep with half the world. I'm finding out pretty much that I have HPV because I've given it to someone else. And, although it's not showing up, I've given it to someone else.

Ingrid felt terrible: "I unknowingly gave it to someone else, and I was the first one he'd had sex with." Her case represents the fact that women can be asymptomatic to the point of having no idea of their infection-status until they confront a sexual partner's accusations.

Summer, 20 years old and a clerical worker at the time of our interview, described a similar experience. She had not noticed her first outbreak of external genital warts when her sexual partner came home from a doctor's appointment and said, "You gave me something." She was "dumbfounded" because this was the first time she had ever considered the fact that she might have an STD. She felt, "like shit—it made me feel horrible." Summer tried to explain that she had been "honest with him," and argued her fidelity: "I haven't been with anyone else." As she reeled from the shock that she likely had an STD, Summer tried to confirm that she had not lost her most significant relationship. She described anxiety over the fact that "he was very unresponsive" and did not want to talk with her about his diagnosis or emotional reaction. As neither one of them had any idea that the virus that caused genital warts could remain latent (asymptomatic) for up to several years after exposure and transmission, both felt confused and angry about how this could have happened.

Francine also had her first outbreak while in a monogamous relationship, long after she believes that she had been initially exposed to herpes.

> It really stunk. It was after [we] got married, and we had been together and been sexually active with each other . . . before the herpes showed up, we had had sex with each other for

about three years, unprotected, just with a diaphragm or pill. And, then I started grad school, and I think maybe the stress of all the new stuff. And, I ended up with this sore right above my clitoris, and I couldn't figure out what it was.

When she went in to her sexual health practitioner, she was told, "Geez, this looks like herpes." Even though her practitioner's hypothesis was pre-diagnostic, Francine "was just in shock." While the official results from her herpes cultures would not be in for several days, "I had to go home and tell [my husband] that I had this outbreak of herpes." She remembered being "really fearful," not because she thought her husband had been unfaithful or "that he would think that I had recently had sex with somebody else." However, she "was still really afraid of what it would do to our relationship because I was devastated by the thought." As Francine's story illustrates, the mere thought that one has an incurable STD can be enough to launch health anxieties and, in cases of having exposed a partner, devastating feelings of guilt.

Woman as the Accuser

The women above were the exception on matters of betrayal, as the majority of the women who experienced betrayal as a component of their initial outbreaks were in the position of having had a partner betray their trust. Having gained reasons to believe that they might have contracted an STD, the women in this sub-group engaged in "retrospective interpretation" (Kitsuse 1962), looking back on their past sexual partners behaviors differently in light of their new experiences.

Most of the women in the position of accuser remembered feeling anger when their STD anxiety prompted them to deduce from whom they might have contracted an infection. For example, Diana, a 45--year-old African American professional, stated that when she began to experience vaginal pain, her first reaction was to see her gynecologist. But, before she received test results that would ultimately confirm genital warts, she called up her ex-partner. After listening to her describe her symptoms he revealed, "Well, you know, my girlfriend had given me some cream for some bumps on my penis." Hearing this information, Diana became "really outraged." She explained, "Basically he had had some kind of an outbreak and had slept with me unprotected, which I just thought was unconscionable. It was like, you know you might have something, and you're gonna' sleep with them anyway!"

Similarly, Kayla, who had contracted Chlamydia and HPV from a boyfriend whose integrity she had doubted, recounted how feelings of betrayal magnified her anxiety of experiencing her first STD symptoms.

> I was pretty upset because he didn't even tell me that he had this, and when I confronted him and told him what I had, he already knew he had a wart and didn't tell me. So he wasn't surprised about that . . . he had already known that he had the warts but hadn't ever told me.

Kayla remembered that she had burst out crying when she absorbed the fact that he had knowingly exposed her to HPV with no regard for her health.

While women like Diana and Kayla had not discussed STDs with ex-partners until after noticing their own symptoms, some of the women had taken precautions to promote honesty and disclosure, yet still fell victim to partners' deceptions. For instance, Ashley, a 21-year-old, white, upper-middle-class undergraduate, thought she had acted wisely by having a talk about sexual history before having sex with a male partner: "He had told me he'd been tested for everything, so I assumed that I was okay." When she "found out later that he was just the biggest liar in the whole wide world," Ashley had already contracted a cervical HPV infection. In addition to feeling "really nervous" when her routine Pap smear came back positive, she also chastised herself for having exercised poor judgment: "I'm a fool, just stupid." Self-degradation like hers often accompanied the role of accuser.

Summer, who had felt guilty for having given her partner genital warts, also traced her infection back to a previous partner who lied about his sexual health status. However, she was also angry with herself because she remembered having seen warts on this partner, confronting him, and believing his answer:

Probably about the third time we had sex, we were lying in bed, and I was fondling him, and I looked over at his penis, and he had these funny little white bumps on his penis. I looked at him and said, "What is that?" And he goes, "Oh, those are just little moles, and I've had 'em since I was a kid." I have a white mole in my armpit, and I'm like, okay. Yeah. That's what that looked like. Sure, but, it still made me uncomfortable, and so I told him, "I don't want us to keep having sex without using condoms until you go and get tested period." And he said, "Well, I've never had anything wrong with me."

Summer, believing that he had had those "little white bumps" examined by a sexual health professional, did not insist on correct and consistent use of condoms.

Ingrid, alerted to her HPV status after finding out that she had likely infected her current partner, told a similar story of having asked for her ex-partner's sexual history. She even went so far as to have "checked out" his penis "with the lights on" as guest speakers in her middle school sexual health class had recommended years before. She relayed the conversation that had occurred after discovering the "bump" on her ex-partner's penis: "I said, 'What's that?' And he said, 'It's been there my whole life.' And I said, 'Are you sure?' He goes, 'It's my penis. I would know.'" Ingrid remembered reflecting back on the middle school slide show presentation from the AIDS organization that had focused on STDs and people of color: She remembered pictures of "herpes and crazy lesions," that did not look at all like what she was seeing on her boyfriend's penis. She explained that this was why she believed his lie. However, when she later contracted HPV, Ingrid insisted on taking the blame for not having known what a genital wart looked like. In her case, I contend that she was betrayed both by a dishonest boyfriend and an inadequate sex education.

The same could be said of Gloria who, as a Catholic Chicana growing up in the 1960s, had received no formal or informal sex education about STDs. When she was 25 years old, she had a sexual partner, and there was "obviously something on his penis," but "it didn't dawn on me that it was something I could catch." At this point in her story she related back to her lack of education: "I mean no one, not even the doctor, after [I had my] children, said anything to me about STDs—I had no idea." So when she worked up the courage and "asked him what it was, and he said, 'Oh, it's nothing; it's something that I was born with," she "didn't think anything of it." That is, until she had her first outbreak of genital warts and experienced a double dose of anxiety over what was happening to her body and how much she had to learn about sexual health.

During the *STD Anxiety* stage, the women had gained reasons to believe that medically 'bad news' was imminent. The myth of *sexual invincibility* had been shattered, as they discovered that they had likely not been immune to sexual health risks. While some of the women had initially tried to deny early signs, growing anxieties motivated all of them to seek out medical care, which lead to them receiving official diagnoses of their illness conditions.

4   The Immoral Patient

nteractionist analyses of illness view diagnoses as dynamic and subjective symbolic representations of illness that take form and change meaning during interactions. This perspective holds that individuals derive self-evaluations by incorporating the perceived evaluations of significant others (Schwartz et al. 1966). In the case of illness, medical practitioners are often the first "significant others" to deliver the possibility of a new identity: That of a sick person. From the patient's point of view, her practitioner's presentation of her STD diagnosis was often the first social interaction to be explicitly impacted by this new, medical identity. As the woman entered this stage, many had their worst fears confirmed and began the process of defining the meaning and probable consequences of their now "official" statuses as sexually-diseased women.

When asked to describe the medical appointments during which they received test results that confirmed diagnoses of genital HPV and/or herpes, the women in my study first recalled different degrees of "diagnostic shock" (Charmaz 2000), depending upon the absence or presence of noticeable symptoms. I then asked them to describe how their perceptions of themselves as sexual beings were affected by these official declarations that something was seriously, contagiously, and incurably wrong with a part of their sexual bodies. The women entering the *Immoral Patient* stage in the sexual-self transformation process had their worst fears confirmed, and they began defining the meaning and consequences of their now "official" status as a sexually-diseased woman.

Utilizing Goffman's (1972) framework, I view the diagnostic encounter as a distinct episode that, as Radley (1994) argued, should be regarded as "a realm that has special meaning, and in which a particular language of reality is binding" (99). This chapter explores the language used and meaning created during diagnostic interactions to reveal how the women define the losses they experienced, as a result of being diagnosed with chronic STDs. Interactions during each STD diagnostic encounter shaped individuals' definitions of illness losses: Losses that manifest as gains in stigma and threats to portions of their identities.

I found evidence that the women experienced all three types of stigma during this stage of their diagnostic encounters: "Abominations of the body . . . blemishes of individual character . . . tribal stigma" (Goffman 1963, 4). Analysis revealed that STD diagnoses forced the women to acknowledge that their health, morality, and social statuses had been corrupted by undesirable medical labels. Similar to the chronically ill men studied by Charmaz (1994), their diagnoses triggered "identity dilemmas," the results of "losing valued attributes, physical functions, social roles, and personal pursuits through illness and their corresponding valued identities" (269).

Abominations of the Body

Whether the individual women walked into their diagnostic appointments having experienced visible/tactile symptoms of an infection, or they were surprised by bad news during routine gynecological exams, all saw these incurable diseases as "physical deformities" (Goffman 1963). Like patients with other illnesses that alter their bodies, "the shared meanings concerning body, body functioning, and body shape [were] visibly demonstrated to be violated or altered" (Kelly 1992, 400). Many of the women described their physical symptoms as "disgusting" and "gross." Even in the cases of internal/cervical HPV, where no warts are visible or tactile to the patient, the idea of warts growing on and in those tissue areas generated various levels of revulsion among the women. In part, their emotional reactions and body identity dilemmas stemmed from fears of what current and future sexual partners would think and feel about their genitalia, which had been ostensibly labeled "abominations" by diagnoses that entailed ruin and contagion.

Experiencing the Spoiled Sexual Body

The women immediately responded emotionally to finding out that their bodies were infected, contagious, and possibly marred by STD symptoms. Their reactions to these revised views of their sexual bodies ranged from perceiving the symptoms as "manageable" to feeling like they had just been struck with a "devastating" illness that had irreparably spoiled their sexual body parts.

Twenty-four felt devastated by seeing, feeling, and imagining how STDs had *permanently* harmed their bodies.[4] Most of these women were horrified by the chronic nature of their infections. Frank (1998) noted that individuals perceive their illnesses as "deep" because of "the certainty that it will be permanent and the fear of this permanence" (197). Gloria, 47 years old at the time of our interview, used this reasoning to explain her initial reaction to being diagnosed with herpes: "I was totally embarrassed—humiliated to think that I had something that was not gonna' go away." Ingrid, a 23-year-old white middle-class undergraduate, similarly described her reaction to an HPV diagnosis: "When I found out about the STD, it was really a slam. I was just like, 'I'm so screwed!' The rest of my life is totally dead." Sierra, 23 years old at the time of the interview, summed up her reaction: "I felt pretty devastated because I knew it was gonna' be there forever." Cleo, 31 years old at the time of our interview, remembered feeling at 19 that her body was "marked for life in some way," a quote that sums up the emotions of those who recalled reeling from the idea that their sexual bodies were permanently damaged.

For many of the women, their practitioners reinforced the idea that their sexual body parts had been permanently ruined. Summer, a Native American clerical worker, remembered the exam when she was diagnosed with genital warts: The most horrible part was the practitioner "explain[ing] to me that it's not curable." Several of these women directly asked practitioners for clarification about the chronic-nature and implications of their diagnoses. Gita, a 23- year-old, single Persian American, admitted that she "freaked out" when she was diagnosed with genital warts and asked her practitioner, "Is this a lifetime thing? Am I gonna' have another [outbreak]?" During this stage, Francine, was not yet a health educator and asked her practitioner questions that exemplify the stress of not understanding long-term health implications: "Does this mean we have to stop having sex? We can't have a baby!" While her practitioner assured her that sexual relations and pregnancy were still possible, he could not soften the emotional blow that she could infect partners and future children (in the case of vaginal deliveries).

Implicit in the incurable nature of these diseases was the long-term responsibility of being contagious. In the case of Violet, 35 years old at the time of the interview, her practitioner's description of the diagnosis had a strong impact:

> Just two weeks ago I went to Planned Parenthood and I talked to the doctor there and he said, "If you've had HPV once, it's in your body. And because it's a virus, there's a 5 to10 percent chance of your partner catching it, even if you don't have any symptoms." I freaked. At point I was like, "This is it! I am just totally tainted for the rest of my life. I've got this evil, awful HPV *thing* in me. I could infect anybody now!"

Haley, a single undergraduate at the time of diagnosis, also remembered being more upset by the idea of infecting others than by the fact that HPV was incurable. When her practitioner told her that she could transmit genital warts to sexual partners, Haley remembered: "That really made me feel bad. What made me feel worse than knowing that I had it was that I had the capability of giving it to somebody else."

The larger contexts of the women's other health and illness experiences also shaped the degree to which they felt that their sexual body parts had been spoiled. Three of the women associated their STDs with mortality. Lily, interviewed at age 41, had previously viewed herself as healthy: "I was the survivor, the one that took care of everyone else." Being diagnosed with severe cervical HPV that would require an in-patient surgical procedure, Lily recalled family members' experiences with disease, hospitalization, and death. Similarly, Tasha, interviewed at age 30, remembered feeling devastated when she internalized a view of her sexual body as spoiled by a cervical HPV infection: "I was really scared 'cause my health was not good before this . . . at that point, in my early 20s, I just assumed I was going to die of cancer." Her history of several non-chronic STDs and reproductive disorders, such as pelvic inflammatory disease, had already threatened her fertility.

Prior sexual health experiences also served to increase the women's perceptions of their STD diagnoses as serious long-term risks to their sexual bodies. "What people know, believe, and think about illness, of course, affects what symptoms they think are important, what is viewed as more or less serious, and what they should do" (Mechanic 1982:16). For these reasons, the women's perceptions of their sexual body parts as having been transformed into "abominations" varied according to their health knowledge.

For example, Amelia, a 26-year-old graduate student, also responded to her cervical HPV diagnosis by worrying about cancer: She had taken "the initiative to find out about" the link between HPV and cervical cancer by conducting her own research on the Internet. Julia, a 50-year-old white professional, received diagnoses of not only genital herpes, but also herpes keratitis, a viral herpes infection of the eye. She left the doctor's office worried about more severe consequences. "I was mostly not even thinking about herpes. I was thinking about losing my eye . . . it was a total nightmare." Upon receiving a herpes diagnosis, Francine recalled others' "horror stories" about genital herpes that made her "immediately" worry about how this disease would impact her "ability to have a healthy child." For Heidi, who had graduated high school in the mid-'80s, health fears of being diagnosed with genital warts were overshadowed by a renewed fear of being HIV positive: She reasoned that if she could get one STD, she might also have another.

In contrast to the above women, the other nineteen women in this study left their diagnostic interactions feeling less stigma of bodily abomination because they felt that their infections were, to some degree, manageable physical conditions. Sandy, an undergraduate from a middle-class family, saw a practitioner who told that her cervical HPV infection was not only treatable but also statistically "normal"—a fact she found very comforting. Elle, a working-class graduate student, had seen a campus doctor who helped her to understand that, while herpes may not be officially curable, it may also not be a symptomatic problem forever. Her case epitomizes comprehensive and considerate diagnostic interactions. Elle's doctor asked if she wanted to be tested for other STDs, so she got the "full screening" at that time.

> We talked about herpes' modes of transmission, and she knew that I had oral herpes because I had come in with a heinous outbreak at one time. So, she said, "You know, it's entirely possible for oral-genital transfer," and my partner at the time did occasionally get oral herpes outbreaks. . . . She gave me the prescription and a little background on how the virus works, and how it's known to burn itself out over time.

Prior knowledge about STDs helped a few women to be optimistic about their diagnoses. For Elle, 32-years-old and bisexual, seeing herself as different from others with herpes helped her. "I'd only known a couple of people in the past who had spoken of their herpes diagnoses, and they typically had tales of woe of being cheated on . . . And, I felt like I didn't mesh with that." The only aspect that was potentially scary to Elle was pregnancy: "I have to admit that it did put a tinge on what if I had an unplanned pregnancy. I thought, boy, would I be having a C-section?" However, this fear was negated for Elle because she did not want children.

Among these women who had been led to believe that their sexual bodies were less *spoiled* than was medically accurate was one exception, Chris. She had researched herpes when her ex-husband had his first outbreak and was able to educate her doctor during their diagnostic interaction when he mistakenly told her "that you couldn't spread the virus when you were asymptomatic." Chris, single and 40 years old at the time of the interview, had seen her ex-husband successfully manage his genital herpes infection with antiviral medications.

Other practitioners fostered a lack of knowledge that served equally (if not genuinely) well in minimizing health fears. Many of these women felt calm after receiving STD diagnoses because their practitioners had not fully explained the chronic nature of the infections. In a few cases, practitioners gave significantly incorrect information about the contagious aspects of the STDs in their diagnostic interactions with patients. Helena, 31 years old and single, was given incorrect and incomplete information about HPV. "There was never any discussion about [HPV] . . . no, 'This is what you should do, this is what you shouldn't do from now on.' There wasn't any discussion like, 'You have this for the rest of your life, and you may get cervical cancer from it.'" She, "almost felt like [the practitioner] was going to treat the warts, and then everything was going to be fine . . . because nothing else was really explained." Molly, a wife and the mother of three young children, had a doctor who left her feeling "okay" about a diagnosis of severe cervical HPV by misrepresenting the sexual nature of the virus. He told her it was "not a problem for men because the virus will live in a nice, warm place in a woman's body, but it just washes off the penis." She left the diagnostic encounter believing the bodily harm was manageable because there was no way that she could have or ever would transmit the virus to her husband. For Jenny, a sexually-active college freshman, her doctor's misinformation about cervical HPV left her with a similar sense of false well-being: "The doctor was like, 'You have a really mild case. You know that you can't get genital warts from this. You can't give a guy genital warts.'"

In several cases, practitioners delivered HPV diagnoses without mentioning that the infection was chronic or sexually transmitted, so this sub-group of women believed their diagnoses to be physically manageable. Prior health research has documented that many HPV patients, "were initially informed that they had a 'virus' or 'condyloma.' The sexual route of transmission and the implications of the disease were not even mentioned." (Keller et al.1995, 358). My data confirm this finding and reveal that, for some of the women, this lack of information enabled them to go into a psychological state of denial during their HPV diagnostic interactions, thus reducing the negativity of their diagnostic interactions.

For example, Cleo rationalized her post-diagnostic denial by implicating her practitioner's resistance to addressing the sexual transmission of the virus: "The way everything had gone was really set up for me to just pretend like it never happened." Hillary, 22 years old and still undergoing treatment for genital warts at the time of the interview, also remembered having been "in denial about it." She explained that her practitioner said, "Your Pap smear is showing HPV but that doesn't necessarily mean you have it." Hillary reasoned, "So, just that one time of telling me it might not be HPV, I convinced myself that it wasn't." Similarly, Helena, "almost felt like [my practitioner] was going to treat the warts, and then everything was going to be fine . . . because nothing else was really explained. Of course I was upset, but I didn't really feel a sense of trauma that I ended up feeling later on." Sloppy interpretation of test results, lack of epidemiological knowledge, and insufficient health education all contributed to these women leaving their diagnostic interactions with a false assessment of their future health risk and current health damage. The above women experienced delayed stigma of bodily abomination; but, as Helena's above quote illustrates, all experienced it eventually.

Regardless of the degree to which the women felt that the physical manifestations of STDs were stigmatizing, more than 75 percent used the adjective "dirty" to describe how they viewed their infected bodies. For instance, Heidi, a practicing Christian, recounted her emotional reaction to being diagnosed with external genital warts: "I felt dirty, gross." Comparing her reaction to that of a girlfriend who had herpes, she believed that these two STDs produced similar reactions:

> There're just a lot of "Oh, gross!" reactions to [herpes and HPV] because there are external indications . . . I mean the thing with warts—people are embarrassed when they have warts on their hands. There's just some stigma about warts, like you're just a dirty person if you get them anywhere. Let alone on you know, private parts!

Heidi's and other women's feelings of "dirtiness" provide the imagery to understand why these STDs inspired crises in how they felt about their sexual body parts.

Body Identity Dilemmas

As Frank (1998) noted, "deep" illness experiences can trigger alterations in identity. I draw on Kelly (1992) to connect awareness of a body damaged by illness to identity transformation: He found that radical surgeries created self-awareness "that these differences are undesirable in themselves and likely to be appraised by others as undesirable" (Kelly 1992, 397). Illness had the power to reframe how individuals identified with regard to their health and appearance. In this manner, the women in my study experienced a range of body identity dilemmas.

While some experienced first-hand "disgust," many experienced the disgust of others toward their bodies, either directly from their practitioners or indirectly by imaging partners' reactions. Summer's story combines both experiences, as her practitioner forced her to view her damaged body. "She gets me this mirror . . . and she's showing me what they look like . . . and, then she walked out of the room, and I'm sitting there and I just start crying." For most of the women, initial messages about their diseased sexual body parts came during interactions with their sexual health practitioners. Twenty-seven of the women described their practitioners ranging from compassionate to matter-of-fact in how they verbally, emotionally, and tactilely interacted with their bodies during the diagnostic examination. While none of these women described feeling positively about their lesions, bumps, or abnormal cells, they expressed feeling some level of reassurance that their bodies were normal within the clinical realm of symptoms for these STDs.

However, the other sixteen women received implicit and explicit negative messages about their infected body parts from practitioners who were judgmental and condemning. For these women, their practitioners magnified the patients' already present concerns about how others would react upon knowing about, seeing, and/or feeling their STD symptoms. In some cases, the women felt that their practitioners were truly disgusted, finding their diseased bodies revolting. For example, Chris, who had scheduled a gynecological appointment because of a painful first herpes outbreak, described her doctor interacting with her as if he were a car mechanic assessing a vehicle whose irresponsible owner had created a horrible problem. Laying down with her feet up in gynecological stirrups that swiveled, the doctor "just looked at my crotch and said, 'Yep, that's herpes,' and sort of *slammed* my knees back together . . . like, 'Let's close this back up,' like a car—slam the hood down! Don't want to see anymore of this one." She also compared her being a woman with herpes to being "Typhoid Mary," the implication that she now identified as having a sexual body that endangered others. In another case of perceived tactile communication of disgust, Julia, 50 years old at the time of our interview, recalled that her doctor had abruptly "pulled back" when he examined her: "Like he didn't really want to touch my leg . . . like I was contaminated merchandise."

Practitioners also verbally expressed negative attitudes toward their patients' sexual bodies. Louise, a 28-year-old from the South, received a harsh HPV diagnosis over the phone. "He was very accusatory . . . like now I was this big pain in the ass for having a bad Pap smear . . . I got him on the phone, and he's like, 'You have cancerous growth all over your cervix: It's everywhere. It's probably HPV. You probably picked it up from some guy." Not only had her doctor described a very significant part of her body as ravaged by cancer, but he had also marked her as promiscuous. Her case illustrates a swift transition from bodily abomination stigma to stigma of character.

The belief that certain illnesses stemmed from deviant behavior has a longstanding place in health care: "It is generally agreed that the idea of disease as deviation from a biological norm dominates medical thinking and practice at the present time" (Lock 2000, 261). In recent decades, U.S. health care practitioners have undertaken professional training geared toward counteracting underlying prejudice and creating practitioners with "neutral" or "objective" views toward their patients. However, research has shown that, "In their encounters with patients, doctors may interpret personal problems and encourage individual behaviors in directions that are consistent with society's dominant ideological patterns" (Waitzkin 1989, 225). Society's dominant ideology has assigned stigma to particular types of patients (e.g. the obese, the sexually diseased, the addicted). As exemplified by these women's recollections, the connection between illness and deviance impacts practitioners' verbal and nonverbal communications with some of their patients.

Blemishes of Character

Mirroring Goffman's (1963) conceptualization of this type of moral stigma, the U.S. ideology of STDs is rife with stereotypes of women with "unnatural passions" and "weak wills," as represented by promiscuity. The social construction of women with STDs as morally corrupt derives from the fact that promiscuity has been tied to sexual health risk: Sexual transmission evokes *blame*, and fear of contagion evokes *dread*. Weitz (1991) contends that the presence of these two emotions in ill individuals often signifies that their moral characters have been damaged. Analysis of the women's self-reported emotions during their diagnostic interactions revealed the prevalence of both blame and dread. The data illustrate a process of how these women learned to view STDs as immoral illnesses and, in turn, how these views shaped their initial attempts (i.e., those during diagnostic encounters) to reconcile moral identity dilemmas.

Lessons on Immorality and STDs

The process of acquiring blemish-of-character stigma with an STD diagnosis begins with the women's histories of being socialized to attach morality to sexual health. In the first stage, *Sexual Invincibility*, these women learned what they should think about STDs, in general, and about women with STDs in particular, via formal and informal educational experiences. "Since definitions of illness are ultimately cultural products, their meanings are influenced by social attitudes and cultural stereotypes" (Grove et al. 1997, 318). How these women perceive these sexual social attitudes and cultural stereotypes shapes the effects of stigma on their moral identities.

When asked what ideas they had about people with STDs during junior high and high school, all of the women described a consistent stereotype exemplified by two of the women. Cleo's high school health teacher had presented STDs as "awful" and "bad," so she "thought that only 'bad' people had STDs." Kayla, a practicing Christian, had learned myths about character blemishes of dishonesty and treachery embedded within stories about sexually diseased women, who lied to their partners about their sexual health statuses and risked infecting them.

Because of religious lessons about sex, many of the women had learned to associate premarital sex and promiscuity with sin. For example, all twelve of the women who were raised Catholic recalled learning that STDs were connected to deficiencies in spiritual "goodness," which manifested as "bad" behavioral choices. As an adolescent, Francine remembered her Catholic-school teacher showing a sex education movie that gave her, "the message that there's something very bad about having sex." She recalled, "That film showed sexuality being a temptation of the devil." In her social construction of sexuality, STDs became the mark of the sinner. As detailed in Chapter 2, Ingrid learned from a nun, her Catholic school teacher in seventh grade, that she "didn't have to worry about STDs because [she was] a good Catholic." Implicit in this lesson was the message that those who contracted STDs were lacking in religious and moral fortitude. Of the remaining 31 women who reported as being raised in variety of faiths, all used derogative adjectives to describe the explicit and implicit lessons from their childhood and adolescence about people with STDs.

Moral Identity Dilemmas

Drawing on Goffman's (1963) terminology, as evidenced above, all of the women were clear about the "virtual social identities"—social characterizations—of women with STDs that had just become meaningful for understanding their "actual social identities." These identities became meaningful because of the attributes they "could in fact be proved to possess" (2). As stigmatized individuals, Goffman would argue that an individual with an STD "tends to hold the same beliefs about identity that we do . . . Shame becomes a central possibility" (1963, 7). The shame these women experienced came from being officially labeled with a disease that has been associated with immorality.

Their individual sexual narratives created the socio-historical frameworks by which they evaluated the moral impact of their diagnoses. Medical sociology research has found that "the extent to which [a patient's] needs interfere with an acceptance of an illness definition" defined that individual's evaluation of their diagnosis (Mechanic 1982, 16). Those women who had previously conceptualized their sexual selves as "moral" interpreted their diagnoses as a more significant blow to their moral identities. In contrast, those who had already come to see their sexual selves as morally "spoiled" by prior stigma perceived STD stigma as merely maintaining, rather than damaging, their moral identities.

Thirty-five of the women saw themselves as having far too limited levels of sexual experience, and, in turn, far too high levels of sexual morality, to "deserve" their infections. Examples of this sub-group of women included Monica, a 21-year-old who had contracted external

HPV as a "technical" virgin (i.e. skin-to-skin transmission occurred without penetrative intercourse), and Ingrid, who contracted cervical HPV from her first sexual partner.

A few of the women verbalized the question of "why me" when they struggled to see themselves as immoral. Helena recalled post-diagnosis emotions and questions: "I just came home from the doctor, and I felt so *dirty*—why was this happening to me?" Rebecca had her first herpes outbreak in her early 50s, having been married for eight years, and felt "shaken up" when she was diagnosed "because all of a sudden, [herpes] did have something to do with me. My first reaction was, 'Who, me?'" Louise remembered receiving her cervical HPV diagnosis over the phone and immediately thinking that she was a "slut." However, she felt confused as to how her behavior could have resulted in this outcome:

> I was like, oh, my God—I have an STD! I haven't had that many sexual partners. I've been fairly careful . . . who could I have gotten it from? I trusted everyone that I slept with: We had conversations. They were monogamous relationships as far as I knew. Everyone I knew told me they were clean.

These women's prior moral identities, based in large part on self-evaluations of their sexual behaviors as morally acceptable, clashed with and created internal conflict over the shift to a new and negative moral status.

In addition to looking to their sexual narratives for answers to how they "earned" this brand of immorality, sixteen of the women described diagnostic encounters with sexual health practitioners, whom they perceived as condemning and having labeled them as immoral during diagnostic encounters. These interactions generated an immediate realization of the demoralizing interpersonal implications of having an STD. Molly experienced one of the most blatant cases of inappropriate moral condemnation by a practitioner during the diagnostic exam. Raised Irish-Catholic, she and her husband had both been virgins on their wedding night, and neither had ever committed adultery. Her doctor never bothered to ask her about her sexual history before joking that she, like most women who had been "so sexually active," had HPV. To defend herself against his moral accusation,

Molly confided to her doctor that she had "only had intercourse with two men in my life," explaining that the person who infected her with HPV could be "either my husband or the rapist." She was upset by, "this unfounded assumption that I'm highly sexually active when I'm not." The logical conclusions reached by this subgroup of women was that if a medical practitioner, who was supposedly trained to be objective, could blithely assassinate their characters, then those beyond the walls of the examination room might dole out even harsher judgments.

In some of these cases, the women perceived their practitioners as doubting both their morality and intelligence. This left the women feeling like their characters had been doubly tarnished. When Jasmine, an upper-middle-class undergraduate, saw a gynecologist for external genital warts she recalled her doctor asking, "Well, you've had unsafe sex?" She remembered feeling "like I wanted to pull out my SAT scores and tell her, 'Just look—I'm not stupid!' . . . Someone in the health field should be objective about it and should be there to help you and to answer questions and not say, 'You've done the wrong thing.'" When Violet, a highly educated and successful engineer, was given an HPV diagnosis, her nurse reprimanded, "You should use condoms," in response to Violet's disclosure that she had many, casual partners for whom she did not know their STD status. To Violet, the clear implications were promiscuity and stupidity for not practicing safer sex: She resented the practitioner's choice to go "off on a moralistic trip." Essentially, these practitioners encouraged their patients to demote their moral identities to those of women who were neither good enough nor smart enough to avoid contracting an STD. Violet and the other women's concerns of being viewed as having poor character reflected larger fears of being socially "reclassified" as belonging to a different and lesser category of women.

Tribal Stigma

Testing for the existence of tribal stigma among women with chronic STDs entailed a conceptual expansion of Goffman's (1963) definition. He delineated the scope of tribal stigma to focus on membership, via *ascribed* traits: "Race, nation, and religion, these being stigma that can be transmitted through lineages and equally contaminate all members of a family" (4). When Tewksbury and McGaughey (1997) argued that tribal stigma can be transmitted, via "tribes" that are organized around achieved traits, they were able to contend that many individuals living with HIV/AIDS also experience tribal stigma because this disease has been linked to membership in deviant subcultures: Intravenous drug users, sex workers, and men who have sex with men. In both of the above works, tribal stigma has been discussed as *interpersonal* phenomena, transmitted via group membership or lineage. A thorough analysis of women's experiences with STD stigma required a theoretical expansion of tribal stigma to also include *intrapersonal* impacts on one's inner feelings.

To claim that the receipt of a STD diagnosis may be a stigmatizing experience for women is to claim that women perceive a unique relationship between the attribute, a chronic sexually transmitted disease, and the negative stereotype, the promiscuous *bad girl* or *fallen woman*. In the U.S., as in many countries throughout the world, sexually transmitted diseases have been socially constructed as symbols of immorality for women and continue to be interactionally constructed as shameful stigma that may reduce girls' and women's social statuses. I contend that the good girl-bad girl dichotomy can be conceptualized as two "tribes" of femininity. Women with chronic STDs are viewed by others and by themselves, via Cooley's "looking glass self" ([1902] 1964), as members of the bad girls tribe. Easily identifiable members include prostitutes, adult film actors, and exotic dancers. However, implicit membership extends to the multitudes of girls and women who have ever been labeled as some variation of "slut" or "tease."

Conceptually, this tribe emerged from analysis of the women's initial constructions of meaning in their STD diagnostic interactions. Also, during interviews, I asked the women to share their memories at different times in their lives (primary school, secondary school, college, etc.) of sexual rumors, gossip, and lore about sexually infamous bad girls and women. The data show that membership in the good girls tribe is fragile, requiring strict adherence to culturally specific gender norms of sexual morality. The women's stories revealed that downward mobility into the bad girls tribe was often accomplished with startling ease. Contracting genital herpes and/or HPV was more than enough to qualify as serious transgressions and threaten these women with tribal stigma at the diagnostic stage in the their moral careers as patients.

"Suzy Rottencrotch" and Other Members of the Tribe

When I asked each woman to recall what she had first learned about sexually diseased women, all shared similar stories. Analytically, I conceptualized this pattern as the definitional building blocks for a gendered experience of tribal stigma. Their early memories of "bad" girls and "fallen" women conveyed distinctly similar imagery and came together to form a stigma theory, "an ideology to explain [the stigmatized individual's inferiority and account for the danger [that individual] represents" (Goffman 1963, 5). The women had assigned traits of promiscuity, dirtiness, low socioeconomic status, and recalled that they were often members of racial or ethnic minorities. As Goffman (1963) noted, stigma theory often incorporates rationalizations of animosity toward stigmatized individuals based on status differences.

The women's agreement on the trait of promiscuity was unanimous. Before contracting HPV, Cleo had believed that "you had to be really promiscuous to get an STD." In high school, Ingrid learned the connection between being a bad girl and having an STD when she befriended a girl who had been "forced into prostitution at age eleven and had contracted several STDs, including syphilis and gonorrhea." As an undergraduate, Tanya had also learned to connect STD-status with being a woman who "slept around a lot." When rumors spread about a female student having herpes, she and others mocked this woman by calling her "STD or VD" and ostracizing her from their social group. In keeping with Lemert's (1962) *dynamics of exclusion*, being shut out from more desirable social groups was another price to pay for membership in this tribe.

Tasha clarified the gendered aspect of promiscuity when recounting the myths she had learned: Men contracted STDs "from wanton women," not vice versa. Diana had grown up in a strict, Catholic, African-American household and confessed to having had a similar attitude as a teenager: "I didn't think that I would ever be around anybody who would have something like that. You know, just kind of scum-of-the-earth people had it . . . like, men who hung out with prostitutes." Hence, the double standard of STD morality: Good men can be infected, but any woman with an STD is a bad woman. Ingrid confirmed the inequity evident in sexual morality standards. She recalled one female classmate in junior high who was not known to be sexually active, but "was considered a slut just because she grew boobs," thus she served as a tease to the unrequited desires of her male peers. Highlighting the gendered nature of this category, she talked about a boy of the same age who was sexually active and positively regarded by peers as "the shit."

Several of the women described racial and socioeconomic dimensions of this tribe. Rhonda, a 23-year-old Cuban American working-class administrative assistant, described how she had conceptualized women with STDs prior to her first herpes outbreak and painted a picture of poverty and substance abuse: "She'd be dirty . . . I would picture somebody who's really skinny, like sickly skinny, and just not clean. She'd probably have cold sores . . . like a crack-head." Jasmine, coming from the standpoint of a privileged upbringing, added an educational component to tribal membership: "People [who get STDs] are dirty or just not as intelligent, you know, not smart enough to be safe." Haley added irresponsibility as a tribal trait: A woman who contracts an STD "isn't responsible, just going out and partying, and not really caring about what they're doing and not watching out for themselves . . . someone who doesn't even know what they're doing half the time." Monica's recollection added a racial dynamic to the conceptualization of this social class of women. Her high school health class featured "teenage mothers" as guest speakers to educate girls about the price of female sexuality. All of these teenaged mothers were African-American or Latina and from economically disadvantaged areas. As a white teenager from a middle-class home, Monica remarked that she felt "removed" from the risk of joining their ranks because these girls were "different in all those ways."

In addition to schools and churches, U.S. military institutions have served to clarify the rules of membership for this tribe. Chris recounted a tale of the infamous "Suzy Rottencrotch," a caricature created by the military to exemplify the sexually diseased women. Her ex-husband had shared with her his experiences with United States military programs on STD prevention. According to him, these programs relied heavily on the legend of "Suzy", a loose woman/prostitute who would tempt men on leave to stray from their "good wives" who were faithfully chaste (and "clean") back home. Chris' example clarified how Suzy and her kind represent a different breed of women, the polar opposite in a moral dichotomy of female tribes: The bad girls versus the good girls (good wives and good mothers).

The "Bad Girls Tribe" and Social Identity Dilemmas

In light of the consistent message that contraction of STDs qualifies girls and women for an unsavory social status, all of the women faced a daunting task of confronting their involuntary membership into this tribe. Many found it difficult to reconcile prior conceptions of their sexual selves with their new social status of being a *bad girl*. Having just been diagnosed with a chronic STD, images and symbolic tales of *dirty women* suddenly became relevant in sorting out to what social tribe they belonged.

Thirty-five women felt that the image of the *bad girl* did not fit their social self-concepts. Hillary, an undergraduate who contracted HPV from her third sexual partner, recalled how in the past she had "just thought [STDs] happened to promiscuous, *slutty* people, you know, that's the big stereotype." Haley described feeling jarred and distracted during her diagnostic encounter, as she struggled with the contrast between whom she thought she was and the type of people she thought contracted STDs:

> I was pretty overwhelmed. Like I kind of not ignored [my practitioner], but I kinda' was still thinking about the fact that now I have something. I have this disease. I have this thing, but I never thought I would get it. I never thought I would be one of those people. And here I am, I have HPV. And that was like the only thing that was going through my head.

In contrast to Haley's surprise, Jenny's cervical HPV diagnosis caused her to reflect on how she could have not seen the STD coming and why she had fooled herself into believing she was one of the "good girls." As the practitioner delivered the diagnosis, "Well, I kinda' felt like a slut. . . . I wasn't thinking that when I got to ten, or however many people I had sex with, that I would look back and be like, 'Oh, my god—I've had sex with ten people!'" Anne, a bisexual graduate student who had had sex with approximately eight men and three women, described experiencing a dissonance of sexual selves:

> I feel kind of slimy sometimes when I think about it. Like only slimy people get things like that, and I don't think of myself as slimy. So it's—yeah. It kind of doesn't fit, in a way, with my whole conception of myself. I never thought of myself as someone who would get a sexually transmitted disease and I definitely didn't. Still it doesn't sit well with my image of myself.

For this sub-group of the women, who had previously viewed their sexual selves as moral and "clean" (healthy), it was mentally and emotionally difficult to reconcile stereotypes of *bad girls* with how they saw themselves as social and sexual beings.

In contrast, eight of the women perceived their diagnoses as minimally stigmatizing with regard to social identity because other sexual traumas had previously "earned" them membership in the *bad girls tribe.* For example, Violet, had survived incest and several sexual assaults that had led her to see herself as "totally tainted" before HPV entered her medical reality. She also saw herself as an "awful slut" who had spent her undergraduate years "sport-fucking," a term she defined as "making guys beg for casual sex." Similarly, Julia viewed "getting raped" as making her "feel a little looser about having intercourse." She thought there was no point in trying to view her sexual self as good, "'cause I've been raped and I'm not a virgin anymore." Having come of age in the early 60s, she had learned that virginity was a requirement for being a "good girl." Violet's and Julia's stories exemplify the double bind for women: Whether one sees herself as the object or subject of sexual trauma the resulting blow to social identity remains the same.

Several of the women claimed agency in having "earned" tribal stigma prior to being diagnosed with an incurable STD. Rhonda, saw herself through her Cuban mother's judgmental eyes as a daughter who had done a "series of bad things," including the Catholic sin of terminating a pregnancy - a crisis that she believed held far greater moral and emotional consequences. She reiterated the stereotype of the "promiscuous slut" and confirmed, "I guess I did see myself that way." Likewise, Amelia reflected on her days as the "school slut" who was always worried about getting pregnant and was not surprised to find out she had contracted an STD. Natasha, a 20-year-old white middle-class undergraduate, also saw herself as fitting the STD stereotype of "someone who'd slept around with a lot of people" and felt like she "deserved" her genital warts infection. All of this subgroup of women viewed their prior social identities as being completely congruous with being at risk for contracting an STD. As these women had judged themselves to be promiscuous and sexually unhealthy prior to receiving an official STD diagnosis, their diagnostic encounters did not add tribal stigma, but merely confirmed their pre-existing membership.

One exception to either of the above sub-groups, Elle, believed that her social identity was only mildly altered. While aware of the stereotype that women with STDs were "skanks," she remarked that STDs were "a probability issue" for anybody having sex. Elle viewed her practitioner as "very normalizing and very optimistic." She believed that her positive perception of the morality and health implications of genital herpes had been strongly shaped by the kind nature and educational stance of her practitioner. Her example points to a question: If diagnostic interactions can neutralize the stigma of body and character normally associated with STDs, then does the patient stand a good chance of being immune to tribal Stigma as well? The challenge to finding an answer would lie in locating more women to interview who shared Elle's experience of having had affirming diagnostic encounters.

At this point in their moral careers as STD patients, most of the women could be categorized as having concealable or *discreditable* stigma (Goffman 1963): By virtue of patient confidentiality, each woman was only explicitly labeled or *discredited* in the eyes of her practitioner. My analysis, however, hones in on their perceptions of stigma, "what the putatively stigmatized think other think of them and 'their kind' and about how these others might react to disclosure" (Schneider and Conrad 1981:35). As such, the women experienced their STD diagnoses as stigmatizing to their bodies, character, and social statuses. In turn, they confronted identity dilemmas of who they were, with regard to their bodies as diseased and contagious, their characters as immoral (both to self and others), and their social statuses as demoted to an unsavory caste of women.

Now that the diagnostic label was permanently a part of their medical records, the women internalized the multiple implications for their present and future sexual selves. As Garfinkel (1956) noted, "the former identity stands as accidental; the new identity is the 'basic reality'" (422). Diagnostic stigma were perhaps most damaging because they inspired the women to abandon most positive conceptualizations of their pre-STD sexual selves.

For example, Ashley, 21 years old and single at the time of the interview, described returning home after receiving a cervical HPV diagnosis. Her words summarized the emotional outlook and concerns shared by many of the women at the end of this stage:

> I just went home, and I thought my life was over. Honestly, I lay down on my bed and wanted to die . . . like [this diagnosis] was my sexuality . . . and I looked up the page [in my sexual health book] on HPV, and there was just a little paragraph and two god-awful photos. I saw the warts, and I immediately thought no one's ever gonna' want to marry me. Nobody's ever gonna' love me. And, [given the possibility of] cervical cancer, I'm never gonna' have kids, and I really wanted to have kids. So I just went AWOL.

A diagnosis had made Ashley and the rest of these women feel, to different degrees, like *damaged goods*. Now, their focus had to switch from the intrapersonal to the interpersonal as they faced the challenge of managing STD stigma in the world beyond the doctor's office.

5 Damaged Goods

The women symbolically became *immoral patients*, during interactions with medical practitioners, and within the context of U.S. social values that connect sexual health and feminine morality. Brandt (1987) contended that interactions with medical practitioners and lay people are the conduit through which STD stigma are reinforced. When the women left their doctors' offices newly diagnosed, they entered a stage of stigma management.

As described in the previous chapter, STD diagnoses radically altered the way all but one of the forty-three women saw themselves as sexual beings. They faced daunting medical, personal, and social realities. Reflecting variations in attitudes and experiences, the women employed different strategies to manage their new stigma. Analysis of their illness narratives reveals a range of ways to cope: (1) denial of stigma, (2) deflection of stigma, and (3) acceptance of stigma. Each stigma management strategy had ramifications for the transformation of their sexual selves.

Stigma Denial

Goffman (1963) proposed that individuals at risk for a deviant stigma are either "the discredited" or "the discreditable." Discredited persons' stigmata are known to others because the affected individuals had revealed their deviant status, or because the deviant traits were not concealable. In contrast, the discreditable could hide their deviant stigma during most social interactions. Goffman found that the majority of those living with discreditable stigma "passed" as non-deviants by avoiding stigma *symbols*, anything that would link them to their deviance. He also noted that many utilized *disidentifiers*, props or actions that would lead others to believe they did not have a deviant identity. Goffman (1963) found that individuals bearing deviant stigma might eventually resort to "covering," one form of which he defined as telling deceptive stories. To remain discreditable in their everyday lives, twenty of the women employed denial-based stigma management strategies: passing and/or covering. In contrast, seventeen of the women revealed their health status to select friends and family members soon after receiving their diagnoses. The remaining six women related that they had inadvertently passed for healthy: they had not yet received an STD diagnosis at the time that they portrayed themselves as uninfected.

Passing

The deviant stigma of women with STDs was essentially concealable, though revealed to the necessary inner circle of health care practitioners and health insurance providers. The women knew that they could rely on practitioner-patient confidentiality. For the majority, passing as "STD free" was an effective means of hiding stigma from others, sometimes, even from themselves.

Hillary, 22 years old at the time of our interview, described how she had initially distanced herself from the reality of her HPV infection by using passing strategies.

> At the time, I was in denial about it. I told myself that that wasn't what it was because my sister had had a similar thing happen, the dysplasia. So, I just kind of told myself that it was hereditary. That was kinda' funny because I asked the nurse that called if it could be hereditary, and she said "No, this is completely sexually transmitted" . . . I really didn't accept it until a few months after my cryosurgery.

Similarly, Gloria, a Chicana graduate student and mother of four, was not concerned about a previous case of gonorrhea she had cured with antibiotics or her chronic HPV "because the warts went away." Out of sight, out of her sexual self: "I never told anybody about them because I figured they had gone away, and they weren't coming back. Even after I had another outbreak, I was still very promiscuous. It still hadn't registered that I needed to always have the guy use a condom."

When the women had temporarily convinced themselves that they did not have a contagious infection, it was common to conceal the health risk with partners because the women, themselves, did not perceive the risk as real. For example, Kayla, a college senior at the time of the interview, felt justified in passing as healthy with male partners who used condoms, even though she knew that condoms could break. Cleo, a 31 year-old mother of a toddler, had had sex with a partner soon after being diagnosed with HPV at 19. "So at the time I had sex with him, yes, I knew but, no, I hadn't been treated yet. That gets into the whole 'I never told him' [about the issue], and I didn't. Part of me thought I should, and part of me thought that having an STD didn't fit with my self concept so much that I just couldn't [disclose]."

Francine, 43 years old and the mother of a fourth-grader at the time of the interview, had never intended to pass as STD-free when she was younger. However, she did not get diagnosed with herpes until after beginning a sexual relationship with her second husband, the future father of her child:

> I think there was all the guilt: what if I bring this on you? So, I felt guilt in bringing this into the relationship. Because he had not been anywhere near as sexually active as I had. So, I started feeling remorse for having been so sexually active during the period of time between marriages. So, I think I always felt a little more guilty because I might have exposed him to something through my actions.

Sarah a 24-year-old, white, upper-middle-class graduate student, expressed a similar fear of having passed as healthy and exposing a partner to HPV. "[He] called me after we'd been broken up and told me he had genital warts. And, I was with another guy at the time, doing the kinda-sorta-condom-use thing. It was like, 'Oh, my gosh, am I giving this person something?'" Even in these cases, where the women unintentionally passed as sexually healthy, they felt guilty when looking back at these interactions.

Several of the women also tried to *disidentify* themselves from sexual disease in their attempts to pass as being sexually healthy. Rather than explicitly using a prop or action that would distance them from STD stigma, the women took a more passive approach. Some gave non-verbal agreement to put downs of other women who were known to have STDs. For example, Hillary recalled one such interaction:

> It's funny being around people that don't know that I have an STD and how they make a comment like, "That girl, she's such a slut. She's a walking STD." And, how that makes me feel when I'm confronted with that, and having them have no idea that they could be talking about me.

Others kept silent about their status and tried, in other ways, to maintain their social statuses of being good girls or moral women. Kayla confessed to employing a charade of words and mannerisms that implied her sexual inexperience: "I guess I wanted to come across as like really innocent and everything just so people wouldn't think that I was promiscuous, just because inside I felt like they could see it even though they didn't know about the STD." Putting up the facade of sexual purity, these women distanced themselves from any suspicion of sexual disease.

Covering

When passing became too difficult, some women resorted to fiction to dissuade family and friends from the truth. Cleo summed up her rationale, comparing her STD cover stories to what she had learned growing up with an alcoholic father. "They would lie, and it was obvious that it was a lie. But, I learned that's what you do. Like you don't tell people those things that you consider shameful, and then, if confronted, you know, you lie."

Hillary talked to her parents about her HPV surgery, but never as treatment for an STD. She portrayed her moderate cervical dysplasia as a pre-cancerous medical scare, unrelated to sex. "We never actually talked about it being a STD, and [my mother] kind of thought that it was the same thing that my sister had which wasn't sexually transmitted." Tasha described how she had initially learned to manage the shame of STDs when she was first infected with "crabs." Her older sister had helped her get a prescription for pubic lice and actually provided the cover story for her embarrassed younger sister. "She totally took control, and made a personal inquiry: 'So, how did you get this? From a toilet seat?' And, I was like, 'yes, a toilet seat,' and she believed me." When I asked Tasha why she confirmed her sister's misconception, she replied, "Because I didn't want her to know that I had had sex." For Anne, 28 years old at the time of the interview, a painful herpes outbreak almost outed her on a walk with a friend. She was so physically uncomfortable that she was actually "waddling." Noticing the strange walking style, her friend asked what was wrong. Anne told her that it was a hemorrhoid. This was a partial truth, but herpes was the primary cause of her pain. As Anne put it, telling her friend about the hemorrhoid "was embarrassing enough!"

Deception and Guilt

The women who chose to deny, pass as healthy, use disidentifiers, or tell cover stories shared more than the shame of having an STD: They had also lied. With lying came guilt. Anne, who had used the hemorrhoid cover story, eventually felt very guilty. Her desire to conceal the truth conflicted with her commitment to being an honest person. "I generally don't lie to my friends. And I'm generally very truthful with people, and I felt like a sham lying to her." Deborah, a 32-year-old from the Midwest, only disclosed to her first sexual partner after she had been diagnosed with HPV: She passed as healthy with all later partners. Deborah reflected, "I think my choices not to disclose have hurt my sense of integrity." However, her guilt was resolved during her last gynecological exam when the nurse practitioner confirmed that, after years of "clean" Pap smear results, Deborah was not being "medically unethical" by not disclosing to her partners. In other words, it could be assumed that her immune system had won the battle against the virus, so she might never experience another outbreak or transmit the infection to sexual partners.[1]

When Cleo passed as healthy with a sexual partner, she started, "feeling a little guilty about not having told." However, Cleo experienced severe consequences for having passed as STD-free:

> I never disclosed it to any future partner. Then, one day, I was having sex with Josh, my current husband, before we were married, and we had been together for a few months, maybe, and I'm like looking at his penis, and I said, "Oh, my goodness! You have a wart on your penis! Ahhh!" All of a sudden, it comes back to me.

Cleo's decision to pass left her burdened with the guilt of deceiving and infecting her husband and the worries of how this might impact their future plans for having children.

Surprisingly, those women who had *unintentionally* passed as being sexually healthy (those who had no knowledge of their STD-status at the time) expressed a similar level of guilt as those who had been purposefully deceitful. For instance, Violet, at 35 years old, had inadvertently passed as healthy with her current partner. Once she received her diagnosis, she disclosed to him, but she still had to deal with the guilt over possibly infecting him.

> It hurt so bad that morning when he was basically furious at me, thinking I was the one he had gotten those red bumps from. It was the hour from hell! I felt really majorly [sic] dirty and stigmatized. I felt like "God, I've done the best I can: If this is really caused by the HPV I have, then I feel terrible."

When employing passing and covering techniques, the women tried to keep their stigma from tainting social interactions. They feared reactions that Lemert (1962) has labeled the *dynamics of exclusion*: Rejection from their social circles of friends, family, and, perhaps most importantly, sexual partners. For most of the women, guilt surpassed fear and became the trigger to disclose. Those who had been deceitful in passing or covering had to assuage their guilt: Their options were to remain in denial, disclose, or transfer their guilt to somebody else.

Stigma Deflection

As the women struggled to individually manage their STD stigma, both real and imaginary social interactions became the conduit for the label of "damaged goods." Now that the unthinkable had happened to them, many of the women began to think of their past and present partners as infected, contagious, and potentially dangerous to themselves or other women. The combination of transferring stigma and assigning blame to others allowed the women to deflect the shame of their illnesses away from themselves.

Stigma Transference

I propose the concept of *stigma transference* to encompass this category of stigma management that has not been addressed by other deviance theorists. To clarify, stigma transference is not a specialized case of projection: "the unconscious process in which the individual attributes to others his or her own emotions and impulses . . . a common defense mechanism, used by the ego to control unacceptable feelings, thereby helping to reduce anxiety" (Marshall 1994, 421). Stigma are neither emotions nor impulses; rather stigma are conceptualized relationships of devaluation (Goffman 1963). When the women transferred their stigma, they attributed their devalued relationship with sexual health ideals to real and imaginary others. Stigma transference strategies manifested as clear expressions of anger and fear. The women did not connect this strategy to a reduction in their levels of anxiety; in fact, several discussed it in relation to increased anxiety.

Cleo remembered checking her partner's penis for warts after her doctor told her that she could detect them by visual inspection. It became a "habit" for Kayla to check her partner for any visible symptoms of an STD. Gloria was more careful about "checking" future partners and asking if they "had anything." Tasha explained, "I just felt like I was with someone who was dirty." In all four cases, the women were only sure of their own STD infections, but, in their minds, they believed their partners to be diseased.

Transference of stigma to a partner became more powerful in cases where the woman felt betrayed by her partner. When Hillary spoke of the "whole trust issue" with her ex-partner, she firmly believed that he had lied to her about his sexual health status and that he would lie to other women. Even though she had neither told him about her diagnosis, nor had proof of him being infected, she fully transferred her stigma to him.

> He's the type of person who has no remorse for anything. Even if I did tell him, he wouldn't tell the people that he was dating. So it really seemed pretty pointless to me to let him know [that I was diagnosed with a STD] because he's not responsible enough to deal with it. And, it's too bad: Knowing that he's out there spreading this to God knows how many other people.

Kayla also transferred the stigma of sexual disease to an ex-partner, never confronting him about whether or not he had tested positive for a STD. In the wake of her diagnosis, she managed her stigma by labeling him as infected and as a "male slut": "I don't know how sexually promiscuous he was, but I'm sure he had had a lot of partners." Robin, 21 years old at the time of the interview, went so far as to tell her ex-partner that he needed to see a doctor and "do something about it." He doubted her ability to pinpoint contracting genital warts from him and called her a "slut." Robin believed that *he* was the one with the reputation for promiscuity and decided to "trash" him by telling her two friends who hung out with him. Robin hoped to spoil his sexual reputation and scare off his future partners. In the transference of stigma, the women ascribed the same auxiliary traits onto their past sexual partners that others had previously assigned to them.

In a different twist, Anne did not transfer her stigma to her partner, as the two of them believed that his previous girlfriend had betrayed his trust:

> He felt terrible about his own infection—he was angry at the woman who infected him because she didn't tell him [that she had genital herpes]. They had a verbal agreement that they were having a monogamous relationship, and then she was not monogamous with him. She infected him with a sexually transmitted disease. And he was just really upset and felt like he didn't want to pass that on. He didn't want to continue that cycle. So then when he infected me, he felt horrible.

Anne's partner had revealed his herpes status to her before they had become sexually intimate. His disclosure, "being so up front . . . before he even kissed me," ended up preventing him from being the target of her stigma transference.

In all cases, it was logical to assume that past and current sexual partners may have also been infected. However, the stigma of being sexually diseased had far-reaching consequences into the imaginations of some of the women. The traumatic impact on their sexual selves led most of the women to infer that future, as yet unknown, partners were also sexually diseased. Kayla summed up this feeling: "After I was diagnosed, I was a lot more cautious and worried about giving it to other people or getting something else because somebody hadn't told me." They had already been damaged by at least one partner. Therefore, they expected that future sexual partners were also likely to be *damaged goods.*

Hillary, who was still dealing with a genital warts outbreak at the time of our interview, no longer found casual sex appealing. She had heard of other men and women who also had STDs, but stayed in a state of stigma denial, never altering their lifestyle of having casual, unprotected sex:

> I just didn't want to have anything to do with [casual sex]. A lot of it was not trusting people. When we broke up, I decided that I was not having sex. Initially, it was because I wanted to get an HIV test. Then, I came to kind of a turning point in my life and realized that I didn't want to do the one-night-stand thing anymore. It just wasn't worth it. It wasn't fun.

At this stage in her sexual-self transformation, Hillary imagined her world of possible partners as having been polluted with contagion.

Anne's lesbian friends introduced her to a theory of selective stigma transference. One friend claimed that her secret to sexual health was to only have sex with female partners. Anne had disclosed her herpes status in a cathartic interaction with a close, lesbian friend. This friend reacted by shouting, "Those rotten men! You should just leave them alone. It's clear that you should be with women, and it's safer and better that way. Women don't do this kind of thing to each other." Her friends' guidance was an overt attempt to encourage Anne to believe that only potential male partners were likely to be infected.

Rather than thinking in terms of sex, Gloria, a Chicana, made a distinction about stigma transference based on ethnicity as a predictor of sexual health status:

> Now, if it was a White man, I made 'em wear a condom because I got it from a White man, and so I assumed that there had to be something with their culture—they were more promiscuous. But, one thing I do know culturally, and with the times, is that Chicano men were more likely to have a single partner.

These women felt justified in their newfound attitudes about sexual partners. What was only supposed to happen to "bad" women had happened to them. Overall, these women transitioned from blaming their own naiveté to blaming someone else for not being chaste, more cautious, or more honest.

Blame

Stigma transference techniques represented the women's attempts to alleviate their own emotional burdens. Initially, the finger of shame and guilt had pointed inward, toward the women's core sexual selves. Their sexual selves became tainted, dirty, and damaged. In turn, they directed the stigma outward to both real and fictional others. Blaming others was a way for these women to alleviate some of the self-blame and turn their anger outwards. Stigma transference allowed them to protect their sexual selves by externalizing the pain of their stigma.

Francine recalled how she and her first husband dealt with the issue of genital warts by re-examining his past as an undergraduate member of a fraternity. "We kind of both ended up blaming it on the whole fraternity situation. I just remember thinking that it was not so much that we weren't clean, but that he hadn't been at some point, but now he was." Francine's first husband had likely contracted genital warts from past sexual activity at fraternity parties: "We really thought of [the HPV] as that woman who did the 'trains' [serial sexual intercourse]. It was still a girl's fault kind-of-thing." By externalizing the blame to nameless women from her husband's past—years of college fraternity, parties—Francine exonerated not only herself, but also her husband.

Similarly, Sarah found a way to blame "the other woman." While internalizing the image of her sexual self as *damaged goods*, she wanted to deflect the blame away from herself. She also wanted to avoid blaming her ex-partner because she was contemplating getting back together with him:

> So, then I thought, "Oh, he was with that floozy, dirty woman before we got back together: The last time." And, then I thought, [the HPV infection] could be latent—for up to 18 months. I'm like, "That falls within the 18-month guideline. It was definitely her." So, I decided it was her who gave it to him, who gave it to me.

For Violet, it was impossible to neatly deflect the blame away from both herself and her partner:

> I remember at the time just thinking, "Oh man! He gave it to me!" While, he was thinking, "God, [Violet]! You gave this to me!" So, we kind of just did a truce in our minds. Like, "Okay, we don't know who gave it—just as likely both ways. So, let's just get treated." We just kind of dropped it.

When faced with an identity-threatening stigma, the impulse to place blame was strong, even when there was no easy target.

The easiest targets for blame were male partners who seemed to have a reputation or *master status* of being "players" and exhibited the *auxiliary traits* of promiscuity and deception. For example, Tasha wasn't sure which ex-partner had transmitted the STD. However, she rationalized blaming a particular ex-partner. "He turned out to be kind of huge liar—lied to me a lot about different stuff. And, so I blamed him. All the other guys were, like, really nice people, really trustworthy." Likewise, when I asked Violet who she believed had infected her with a curable STD, she replied, "Dunno', it could've been from one guy, because that guy had slept with some unsavory women, so therefore he was unsavory." Later, Violet contracted HPV, and the issue of blame contained more anger: "I don't remember that discussion much, other than being mad over who I got it from: 'Oh it must have been [him] because he had been with all those women.' I was mad that he probably never got tested. I was okay before [having sex with] him." The actual guilt or innocence of these blame targets was secondary. What mattered to the women was that they could hold someone else responsible for their STDs.

Stigma Acceptance

Eventually, every woman in the study stopped denying and deflecting the truth of her sexual health status. At the point when each decided to own up to the truth about their STD, the women shifted strategies and began to manage their stigma by disclosing to loved ones. The women disclosed for either *preventive* or *cathartic* reasons. That is, they were either motivated to reveal their STD status to prevent harm to themselves or others, or to gain the emotional support of confidants (Adler and Adler 2006, 290).

Preventive and Cathartic Disclosures

The decision to make a preventive disclosure was linked to whether or not the STD could be cured. Kayla explained, "Chlamydia went away, and I mean it was really bad to have that, but, I mean, it's not something that you have to tell people later 'cause you know, in case it comes back. Genital warts, you never know." Kayla knew that her parents would find out about the HPV infection because of insurance connections. Prior to her cryosurgery, Kayla decided to tell her mom about her condition:

> I just told her what [the doctor] had diagnosed me with, and she knew my boyfriend and everything, so, it was kind of hard at first. But, she wasn't upset with me. Main thing, she was disappointed, but I think she blamed my boyfriend more than she blamed me.

For those women who had close relationships with their parents, it was common for parents to blame their daughters' ex-sexual partners.

Preventive disclosures to sexual partners, past and present, were a more problematic situation. The women were choosing to put themselves in a position where they could face blame, disgust, and rejection. For those reasons, the women typically put off preventive disclosures to partners as long as possible. Anne admitted that she would not have disclosed her herpes to a female sexual partner had they not been, "about to have sex." In Cleo's case, she told her partner about her HPV diagnosis because she wasn't going to be able to have sexual intercourse for a while after her cryosurgery. Violet described her thought process that culminated in a decision to disclose her HPV status to her current partner:

> That was really scary because once you have [HPV], you can't get rid of the virus. And, then, having to tell my new partner all this stuff. I just wanted to be totally upfront with him: We could use condoms. Chances are he's probably totally clean. I'm like, "Oh my god, here I am tainted because I've been with, at this point, 50 guys, without condoms. Who knows what else I could have gotten?" (Long pause, nervous laugh) So, that was tough.

For Summer and Gloria, their preventive disclosures were actually a relief to their sexual partners. Summer decided to disclose her genital warts to a new boyfriend after they had been "getting hot n' heavy." Lying in bed together, she said, "I need to tell you something." After she disclosed, he lay there, staring at the ceiling for a couple of minutes before exhaling deeply and saying, "I thought you were going to tell me you had AIDS." Similarly, one of Gloria's partners sighed in relief when she revealed that she had herpes; he thought she was going to tell him that she was HIV-positive.

The women related many cathartic disclosures with family members. They were motivated to disclose because secrecy had become a burden, they felt vulnerable and wanted the support of those who had known them the longest. Having reached a point in managing their stigma where they were willing to risk criticism, each recalled hoping for positive outcomes: Acceptance, empathy, sympathy, or any form of nonjudgmental support. Tasha's first STD disclosure involved her earlier Chlamydia infection:

My family died laughing: "Guess what, mom, I got Chlamydia."
She's like, "Chlamydia? How did you find out you got Chlamydia?" I'm like, "Well, my boyfriend got an eye infection."
(laughter) "How'd he get it in his eye?" (laughter) So, it was the
biggest joke in the family for the longest time!

Tasha felt that her family's good-natured teasing was a sign that they
were open to talking about STDs. She explained how this positive disclosure experience made her feel more comfortable when, a few years
later, she told her family members about her HPV infection.

However, not all women felt comfortable disclosing their sexual
health status to all family members. Rebecca, a white professional in
her mid-fifties, shared her reasoning for *not* disclosing to her adult
children. "I wanted to tell my younger one . . . I wanted very much for
him to know that people could be asymptomatic carriers because I
didn't want him to unjustly suspect somebody of cheating on him . . .
and I don't believe I ever managed to do it . . . it's hard to bring something like that up." Part of her reluctance to disclose may have been
concerns that her son's view of her would change: He may have had
difficulty reconciling his image of his mother with images of the type
of women likely to contract herpes.

Rather than risk delicate familial relationships, the women often
unburdened their feelings of shame and guilt onto their close friends.
Cleo shared her post-diagnostic concerns with her female roommate:
"I told her that I was feeling weird about having had sex with this second guy, knowing that I had an STD." Kayla's cathartic disclosure with
her best female friend ended up being reciprocal. "At that time, she
was also going through a similar situation with her boyfriend, so I felt
okay finally to talk about it." Deborah only disclosed to "a handful" of
female friends, never to any male friends. She felt that her male friends
would have been more likely to judge her. In Anne's case, her cathartic
disclosure to a female friend was twofold: Both to seek support and to
apologize for initially having used the hemorrhoid cover story. Anne
explained to her friend that she had felt too uncomfortable to originally tell her the truth. "Later, when I did tell her the truth, I was
embarrassed and said, 'I need to tell you that I wasn't completely honest with you before.'" While the majority of the women felt more comfortable confiding in female friends, Lily, a single parent of a teenaged

son, disclosed to a male friend and found relief when she shared her fears about what was happening to her. This male friend was able to be both "emotional and supportive."

Consequences of Disclosure

With both cathartic and preventive disclosures, the women experienced some feelings of relief in being honest with significant people in their lives. However, they still carried the intense shame of being women infected with contagious and incurable sexually transmitted diseases. This combination of feelings—both relief and shame—culminated in anxiety over how their confidants would react: Would they face rejection, disgust, or betrayal? Francine was extremely anxious about disclosing to her current (second) husband. "That was really tough on us because I had to go home and tell [him] that I had this outbreak of herpes." When asked what sorts of feelings that brought up, she immediately answesred: "Fear. You know I was really fearful—I didn't think that he would think I had recently had sex with somebody else . . . but, I was still really afraid of what it would do to our relationship." Hillary's anxiety over revealing her deviant status to strangers almost prevented her from taking advantage of a sexual health support group:

> I think one of the biggest fears for me was walking into a support group and seeing someone that I knew there. But then I turned it around and decided that they were just as vulnerable as I was . . . but, I think the biggest part was just having people find out about what I had.

Even though the other women in the support group would have shared the stigmatized status of sexual infections, each participant represented a potential gossip.

Overall, disclosure strategies intensified the women's anxieties of having their secret leaked to unknown others, in whom they would have never chosen to confide. In addition, each disclosure brought with it the possibility of rejection and ridicule from the people whose opinions they valued most. For Gloria, disclosing was "the right thing to do" but had emotionally painful consequences when her partner's condom slipped off in the middle of sexual intercourse: "I told him it doesn't feel right. 'You'd better check.' And, so he checked, and he just jumped off me and screamed, 'Oh fuck!' And, I just thought, oh no, here we go. He just freaked and went to the bathroom and washed his penis with soap. I just felt so dirty."

The risk of disclosure paid off for Summer, whose boyfriend asserted, "I don't ever want to be *that guy*—the one who shuns people and treats them differently." He borrowed sexual health education materials from her and spent over an hour asking her questions about various STDs. Even with this best-case scenario, the sexual intimacy in this relationship became problematized (e.g., having to research modes of STD transmission and safer-sex techniques). Disclosures were the interactional component of self-acceptance. The women became fully grounded in their new reality when they realized that significant people in their lives were now viewing them through the lens of sexual disease.

Initially, most of the women tried to deny a new, deviant health status that was already protected by healthcare practitioner/patient confidentiality laws. While many used passing and covering techniques that relied on deception of others, self-deception was impossible to maintain. In order to strategize a successful ruse, it was necessary to know the scope of what they were trying to hide. The medical truth began to penetrate their sexual selves as soon as they consciously fabricated their first lies.

When guilt caught up with them, making it hard to pass as healthy, their goal shifted to stigma deflection. Those who engaged in stigma transference imagined forcing "blamed others" to look into the same mirror of judgment which they, themselves, faced. However, deflection only delayed the inevitable: A deviant sexual self that threatened to overtake the women's prior conceptions of themselves as sexual beings.

After mentally transferring their stigma to real and imaginary others, all of the women finally accepted their tainted sexual health status via the reflexive dynamics of disclosure. Voluntary disclosure to intimate others took their sexual health status out of the doctor's offices and into their lives. Each time they told their story to a friend, family member, sexual partner or ex-partner, the women revised the story of who they were as sexual beings. These new stories gained veracity in the verbal and non-verbal responses of the trusted few. Adjusting to the images of themselves reflected in their loved ones eyes, their "looking glass selves" (Cooley 1902/1964) merged with their views of themselves as *damaged goods*. The women's sexual selves moved along a deviant "career path," via the interactive dynamics of their stigma management strategies.

6 Sexual Healing

The women's needs to manage the stigma of having an incurable STD frequently preceded the actual start of medical treatment. However, the issue of stigma management was not necessarily resolved prior to receiving treatment. In this stage of their illness trajectories, the women turned to medical experts for relief and guidance. Cline (2006) cautioned that "even if patients are able to seek care in their communities, the issues of stigmatization, confidentiality, and cultural differences make STD care particularly challenging for providers and patients" (355). Part of *sexual healing* included the women's struggles to understand the line between what treatments could offer in the way of physiological relief and what remained untreatable aspects of having a chronic, contagious infection.

Treatments for genital herpes and HPV came with no guarantees. Caveats as to effectiveness, risk, and pain accompanied the variety of treatment options available. Patient-practitioner power discrepancies often added to the stress of selecting and complying with treatment plans. In addition, the pain of treatments and feelings of anger over lost sexual health status taxed the women's emotional strength. To endure the ambiguity of their healing process, the women struggled to reconcile the reality—that there would be no total cure—with their prior conceptions of themselves as sexually healthy.

Frank (1991) posed a question that plagues the treatment stages of those with serious illnesses: "If recovery is taken to be the ideal, how is it possible to find value in the experience of an illness that either lingers on as chronic or ends in death?" Broad questions, such as this one, and specific questions about their infections, guided the women's search for answers as they focused on the issue of recovery. However, interactions with healthcare practitioners and health education resources served to gradually revise their definitions of "ideal" treatment outcomes.

Negotiating Practitioner Relationships

Receiving treatment for chronic STDs required multiple visits with sexual health practitioners. Unlike previous medical encounters that did not typically require the establishment of a meaningful relationship with a practitioner, the women's treatment plans created situations in which both the medical expertise and bedside manner of their practitioners became highly relevant.

Bedside Manner

Approximately two-thirds of the women described feeling dissatisfied with their practitioners' bedside manners. Louise, who had received notification of an abnormal Pap smear six months after the fact, saw this same practitioner for her initial colposcopy, a procedure that would check for the extent of her cervical HPV infection.[1] She described it as "a horrible experience":

> It was one of those stainless steel rooms, and it was really cold. And I had to wait there for a while before [the doctor] came in. He was very sort of accusatory, you know, maybe because he was defensive [about the delayed results]. He just acted like now I was this big pain in the ass for having had a bad Pap smear. And he wasn't at all nice about it.

Louise's dissatisfaction with her practitioner's lack of compassion paralleled Jasmine's experience of having external warts removed. Jasmine described the treatment when her practitioner applied a topical acid-solution to burn off the warts:

I remember her saying, "It's going to be painful." Like, [she might as well have said] "You deserve this." I felt like she was telling me that this was my punishment. . . . It's just such a hard thing to find out you have a STD, and it's hard to call the doctor and say, "Listen, I need to get treated for this." When I had to go back for two more treatments, I felt like she was disgusted with me, and that hurt worse.

These two descriptions of treatment interactions represented how practitioners' demeanors could increase the difficulty of receiving treatment.

Further examples include cases of women whose practitioners condemned the moral characters of their patients. Janine's recollections of treatment for herpes illustrated the potential for practitioners to explicitly cast moral judgments upon their patients. She worked with preschoolers to supplement her graduate assistantship and found herself feeling "really filthy being with these children because [my second] outbreak lasted forever." Her practitioner had not prescribed her any medication to alleviate symptoms at her diagnostic exam, so she went back to request treatment:

I had no cream. I still don't know what to use . . . So, I went in, and I just told him I was really having a hard time dealing with this, and that I didn't know who to talk with about it. And he told me that I needed to turn to religion, and that he sees people every day with cancer and [my herpes infection] was just no big deal.

In addition to minimizing her pain and confusion, her practitioner had essentially prescribed a change in religious attitudes as a way to mediate symptoms. She remembered thinking: "I don't believe in God. It's none of his business. I was so outraged that he could, as a medical professional, tell me to turn to religion. If I wanted to do that, I would do that, but I thought it was really not his place." Poor bedside manners made the inherent unpleasantness of treatment experiences much more difficult to bear. Jasmine summed up: "I think, had there been more compassion. or just maybe more listening, [getting treated] would have been a little easier."

While my sample had a socioeconomic bias toward the middle-class, a few of the women noted how they had experienced a relationship between their social class status and quality of care. Pam, whose economic circumstances had fluctuated from middle-class to poverty, hypothesized that socioeconomic status played a role in the disparate quality of care she had received. When she "could afford private health care," she experienced excellent bedside manner: Her gynecologist "made it easier: I remember he sang along to the music during the cryo [sic]—the nurses and I were all giggling. They let me lay on the table afterwards until I felt ready to leave." However, when her "economic situation left me to public health care," she experienced impersonal practitioners who rushed her in and out of procedures.

One-third of the women described practitioner treatment interactions like Pam's former experience, in which practitioner demeanor positively affected their experiences. For example, Haley, 22 years old at the time of the interview, thought her doctor "was really cool," during her appointment for cryosurgery.

> She took me into like her real office, like the room with her desk and all her stuff with the chair in there, with the curtains and stuff like that, so that helped a little bit [before the procedure] . . . I was like on and off crying, just upset—didn't know how it was gonna' feel. She explained to me what [HPV] was, and essentially it was like wart tissue on my cervix and they're going in there freezing it.

Having her practitioner take the time to explain the nature of her infection, and the purpose of treatment, in comfortable, non-clinical surroundings helped Haley to feel more at ease. For the same type of procedure, Amelia, who had done her own research, saw a practitioner who took a less traditional approach, using a mirror to show her what her cervix looked like before and after "it was frozen." She remembers, "at first I didn't really want to see it." But after seeing it post-cryosurgery, she remembered thinking, "it was really neat—it was like a snow-cone." Allowing her to see what had been done to her body helped Amelia to understand the process. She also appreciated that her practitioner, "was talking to me the whole time" in which the procedure took place.

Patient Education

The level of health education offered and provided by practitioners also played a key role in shaping the women's perceptions of their treatment interactions. Clinical health researchers on HPV provide the following advice to practitioners (Keller et al.1995, 360):

> It is also essential to include education/counseling as part of all regularly scheduled follow-up visits. Questions and concerns often arise over time. For example, new questions about transmission, recurrence, and long-term consequences of HPV often come up during follow-up visits. Some issues that need to be assessed are (a) the consequences of having HPV infection, including its impact on daily life, relationships, and self-perceptions; (b) the nature of the support system available; and (c) the client's informational needs.

While these guidelines reflect the optimal level of patient education and counseling, the women's treatment narratives revealed a wide range of experiences.

Several of the women interacted with practitioners who came close to meeting all of their needs and expectations. Kelly, a 31-year-old graduate student, recalled positive educational experiences from a female-male doctor team, beginning with the punch biopsies that would determine the extent of her cervical HPV infection:

> They had the male doctor do the colposcopy to look at it more and take more of a sample—those little circle samples that they do. . . . They were real young doctors, really nice, I liked them both. And they did that and that went fine. I remember they walked me through everything. He would tell me, "You might feel some cramping: this might hurt a bit." And they were all terribly sorry that this was happening. Just, "We're so sorry this has happened. We hope it gets better. It's not serious."

These practitioners referred Kelly to another doctor because the biopsies revealed that her initial diagnosis of cervical HPV had to be upgraded to "severe dysplasia—inside and outside the cervix": Her cervical cells showed abnormalities that are often the precursors to cancer. Her new doctor determined that the best treatment was also the "most aggressive surgery—a cone biopsy." Kelly, only 24 years old at this time, was also HIV-positive and appreciated this doctor's concern for her fertility:

> He said, "I want to be aggressive, I want to get all the diseased cells out of there," but he also said, "I'm still going to try to be as conservative as possible, realizing you're a woman of childbearing age, and you might want to have children down the road." . . . I think every other doctor would have just assumed, "We can cut anything out of her—she can't have children because she's HIV-positive. Thinking about that now that I'm trying to have children, I feel so lucky that I had a doctor who didn't judge me.

Kelly went into the cone biopsy procedure feeling well educated about both the procedure and her doctor's intentions.

Summer, who could only afford to see student doctors at a university hospital, also felt that she received compassion and education during her treatment for her external genital warts. She recalled how her female practitioner alleviated some of her abomination of the body stigma with education about the severity of her HPV infection:

> I was always so embarrassed because [the warts] just seemed so big and gross. And, [my practitioner] says, "Honey, I've seen women that have to have them surgically removed where they block parts of their body." She's explaining this to me, and it makes me feel not as bad.

In addition to sharing anecdotal experiences to alleviate some of Summer's disgust with her body, this practitioner also shared some practical advise on how strengthening a body's immune system can reduce the negative impact of viral infections such as HPV and herpes:

> She says, "What I've discovered and what I've seen that works best is to stop smoking." At the time I was smoking cigarettes again. She said, "Smoking is really bad for you when you're try-

ing to make [the warts] go away." She says something in the nicotine causes the warts to just thrive on it.

This advice complemented Summer's own research on HPV, which included a quarterly publication put out by the American Social Health Association:

> I'd been reading articles in *HPV News*, and the more that I read about it, it seemed like the easiest way women conquered it and kept it from breaking out and making the breakouts go away was just to improve their lifestyle: Eating habits, emotional stress, all of those things.

Summer's story exemplifies how practitioners can serve as a source of new information and confirmation of information patients had already gathered.

For other women, their practitioners provided education about viral latency and helped their patients to sort out from whom they might have contracted the virus. In one case, Tanya, a 27-year-old graduate student, had a practitioner explain to her the probably trajectories of herpes infections:

> One thing that she said was that because I hadn't had sex in a while, that generally if you're gonna' break out you break out within the first few months. If you're gonna' stay dormant, you just stay dormant. So she kind of had the idea that [I had contracted herpes] from my current boyfriend . . . especially since we have had unprotected sex.

This explanation helped Tanya to feel better about disclosing to her current boyfriend because she had some medical assurance that he may have been the one to infect her. She felt that this knowledge would help her to counter his possible accusations of infidelity. When it came to treatment, Tanya also felt very satisfied with her practitioner's explanation of how to correctly use both a prescription for anti-viral pills and a topical cream.

Practitioners who played an educational as well as clinical role often worked to create rapport with their patients. Monica described how her practitioner took several treatment sessions to help her better understand how she, as a "virgin," might have contracted genital warts. At her first treatment appointment, she and her practitioner discussed Monica's idea that she had contracted HPV from a toilet seat incident: "That first time, I was in shock. [My practitioner said], "Well there's very, very, small chance that it could be from a toilet seat." Because I couldn't fathom that, she said it's probably not." The practitioner did not force Monica to confront the more anxiety-provoking possibility that the man who had attempted to rape her passed on the virus, via non-penetrative contact. By the time of her second treatment appointment, Monica had "had time to think about it and had more questions going back, once I like had relaxed:" At this time, the practitioner commented, "Yeah, you seemed shocked. I can understand." Then, she proceeded to talk about the more likely routes of HPV transmission and gave Monica "packets on everything they had in the clinic."

Not all practitioners interacted as both healers and educators. Some of the women described practitioners who neglected to explain terminology relevant for a patient's comprehension of both her condition and treatment plan. For example, when Louise went in for her colposcopy, not only did she experience poor bedside manner, her practitioners "didn't tell me anything . . . they just said, 'You know, you have abnormal cells—we're going to do a colposcopy.' I didn't know what that was—I had to look it up."

Some of the women tried to ask for clarification only to be met with defensiveness or distance. Lola, whose European mother had raised her to be open about sexual issues, discovered her practitioner's disappointing attitude toward patient education when she asked his opinion on research she had done:

> When I told him about the research that I had done on the Internet, he got really, really defensive, and he became really agitated. He started just passing over it, saying, "Well, you can't trust what you read on the Internet because that's not regulated, and anybody can post anything on the Internet." It's like he was kinda' making excuses for the information that I found out about my condition. Now I don't know if it was because he felt bad that he didn't tell me these things.

Lola had discovered important and medically accurate information that helped her to better understand the ramifications of her cervical HPV infection and the pro's and con's of the treatment options her practitioner had proposed.

Molly, a nontraditional undergraduate student at 43, described her practitioner as displaying a similar attitude. Due to this, she felt emotionally conflicted about her practitioner interactions during treatment: "I love my doctor. I don't have trouble with my doctor. It's just that there seems to be this impasse or gap that I can't cross." Feeling unable to get answers to her questions, Molly attributed her doctor's stance to a general lack of knowledge about HPV. "There's a lot that's not known: It's better not to suggest that there is fact when there's not fact, and so he tells me they don't know." While she claims to accept his lack of access with regard to education, she also views his attitude as that of "a very clinical, sexist guy who will give you facts if he has them, but if he doesn't have them, he doesn't want to suggest that he does." She used the term "sexist" because she believed that he would treat male patients with more consideration.

Unfortunately, Molly's practitioner was not only reluctant to give her "facts," he also gave her some significantly incorrect information. He told her that medical researchers, "don't know a lot about HPV, but it could be sexually transmitted." As noted in Chapter 4, her doctor had also assured her that the virus could not "live" on men's genitalia. This misinformation left her feeling that she did not have to use condoms with her husband: "They never said that there was any problem with [me] infecting my husband."

A few of the women stood up to intimidating practitioners by insisting on being educated in addition to receiving treatment. For instance, Sierra, in her early 20s at the time of treatment, felt intimidated by both her practitioner's attitude and the dynamics of the clinic, with regard to getting her questions answered about her external genital warts. However, she did not let these factors dissuade her:

> I asked her a ton of questions . . . I'm like, "So, am I gonna'
> have breakouts all the time? Is this something I'm gonna' have
> to like come in to you for [treatments] constantly? If I have it
> on my labia, does that mean I have it on my cervix—how does
> it work? What are my chances of cervical cancer?"

She discussed how if she had not been assertive, then she would have left that appointment undereducated about her condition.

> I was drilling her, but I think if I hadn't been asking her the questions, she wouldn't have answered them because I felt like that doctor's office is so overcrowded, and they have appointments like backed up, that they don't spend the time to educate people. And I was really bummed—I was really disappointed because I just felt like she didn't care that I was her patient. It was like I was someone that she was there to take care of and she was like, "Oh, I guess I can do it."

While Sierra felt "totally brushed off" by her practitioner, her assertiveness paid off in having been able to find out some crucial information. However, when Sierra went in for her three-month follow-up Pap smear, she found out that her practitioner had misled her about one important piece of information: She could still transmit the virus to her sexual partner after treatments for external warts because a Pap smear does not check all cervical tissue for cellular abnormalities. Sierra told her practitioner that she was "disappointed I didn't know that because I've been with [my partner] since [my last Pap smear came back negative] without a condom. I thought I was safe from giving him that and we were protected, you know, because we'd been tested." Sierra recalled that her practitioner responded by being "defensive about it."

Presentation of Treatment Options

The women also faced challenges when trying to have a voice in understanding and selecting their treatment options. A few, like Amelia, sat down with their practitioners and discussed the advantages and disadvantages of different treatment plans. Like Lola, she had done some research on her own and came to her appointment favoring laser surgery for her cervical HPV infection:

> I went to talk to [my doctor] and concluded that if I wanted to do laser surgery versus cryosurgery, then they don't do that [at this clinic]. Laser's also a lot of money . . . I asked her some questions

about what she thought about the different procedures, and she said she thought cryosurgery was the best option.

Amelia was also concerned about testing options for her partner: "I talked to her a little bit more about [what my partner] should do, and she said that there's not a good test and just look to see if there're any warts." In addition, Amelia asked her practitioner what she would do if she had this infection.

> She actually did tell me that it's not scientifically proven, but that some people can take beta-carotene and folic acid after the procedure, that it's a good idea. And she told me that she had had cryosurgery, and she had actually taken those [vitamin supplements], and she told me how much to take of each.

Amelia's practitioner not only welcomed a discussion of different treatment options, but also provided nutritional guidance on how to strengthen the immune system to insure better post-treatment outcomes. Given this pre-treatment interaction, Amelia felt confident and comfortable pursuing cryosurgery.

Unfortunately, the majority of the women encountered practitioners who viewed selection of treatment as a medical decision, not one which involved the patient's input or understanding. Heidi, a working-class graduate student, had a practitioner who did not ask her if she "wanted [the genital warts] burned off or frozen off." She recalled:

> It wasn't until later that I realized I didn't really need to go through that pain right then and there. There were other options . . . I guess it wasn't until after the fact that I realized [my practitioner] didn't really give me an option: She didn't give me a lot of information about it. It was just kind of like, "Oh, I see this all the time. This is what we do. Here you go. Here's a pamphlet. Bye-bye."

Heidi clarified that she did not feel that her practitioner was "judgmental or cold," but rather that she totally excluded Heidi from this decision-making process.

Some of the women dealt with this type of practitioner by being assertive. Ingrid tried to convince her practitioner to perform a colposcopy, the only procedure that could check for the actual extent of her HPV infection. As quoted in Chapter 3, Ingrid had initially discovered her HPV infection because a sexual partner had an outbreak of genital warts, and he had never had skin-to-skin genital contact with anyone prior to being with her. A sexual health educator had recommended she have a colposcopy, so that she could be accurately diagnosed and evaluated for possible treatment options:

> I called [the practitioner] and said I want a colposcopy. She said, "You need a Pap. If I give you a Pap and something comes up, then I'll give you a colposcopy." And I said, "Can things show up on the colposcopy that won't show up on the Pap?" She said, "No, and most insurance companies won't pay for a colposcopy." And I said, "So, if there's nothing wrong with my Pap, then a colposcopy is not necessary?" And, she said, "Yes."

As her attempt to negotiate her needs and clarify her understanding of treatment options with her practitioner had failed, Ingrid added the fact that she knew she had had sex with an infected partner:

> I said, "I had sex with someone who had a genital wart on the head of their penis." And she goes, "Well then, you probably have it. Everybody who comes in here has it because 80 percent of the sexually active population has it. A lot of people have it, but they just don't know it. It's not that big a deal." . . . I was frustrated that she was not updated: I mean she seemed to think that colposcopy wouldn't show anything that the Pap couldn't . . . She also treated my concern of it as not a big deal because everybody has it . . . like get out of my face.

Ingrid left this interaction further convinced that she had HPV and at a loss as to how to go about having her infection assessed and discussing treatment options. In this case, the practitioner was not only wrong with the assessment that a Pap could detect HPV as well as a colposcopy, but she also showed total disregard for her patient's desire to make an informed decision about treatment options. The practitioner's attitude in Ingrid's story illustrated the control maintained by practitioners in the selection and administration of medical treatments (Waitzkin 1989).

Sometimes, the women interacted with practitioners who not only acted autonomously, but also performed treatments incorrectly. For instance, Diana had gone in several years ago to have a sizeable genital wart removed, and her doctor "just sort of cut it off, but there was still a little piece hanging." With HPV, any infected cells that remained meant the possibility of new wart growth.[2] Dissatisfied and feeling that this *scissors excision* treatment had been inadequate, she switched gynecologists and received a different and more effective treatment for her infection: "My current gynecologist thought that's not the way to do it, and he put some kind of acid on it." Her previous doctor had neither presented alternative treatment options, nor carried out the chosen option correctly. Like many of the women, Diana trusted her instincts and found a practitioner whom she could trust to communicate with her and explain treatment selection.

Some practitioners acted autonomously, not only in deciding what treatments to provide, but also with regard to the manner in which services were provided, as well as after-care. Molly, who had described her doctor as "a very clinical, sexist guy," commented on how he and his staff ignored her anesthesia concerns prior to, and her physiological needs after, a cone biopsy:

> I was really terrified about being put under, and, at that time, they did a general [anesthesia]. I was not excited about that at all. But, he said that's the only way he would do it. So I had to have it done. As I could do it on an outpatient basis, they were getting ready to release me, but I was still quite under the effects of the anesthesia. To make a long story short, I got up, and I fell, and it was major: I broke my nose and had a serious cut on my lip and had to have more anesthesia and more surgery . . . my body had never had those drugs before, so it was really wiped out. . . . I fell, so then they had to do second surgery, and I had to be in the hospital for the weekend.

In what could have been considered a case of malpractice, Molly felt that her health care providers had rushed her to stand up, so that she would leave the operating room and free it for the next patient. She remarked on possible ulterior motives: "I'm sure it was driven by the insurance, you know, getting people out of there."

Negotiating the Demands of Treatment

Whether their practitioners alleviated or exacerbated the negative aspects of treatment decisions, the women still had to face the physical, emotional, and financial demands of treatment procedures. Health researchers have noted the burden placed on individuals seeking treatment for chronic sexually transmitted diseases: "STDs, such as herpes and venereal warts, require a lengthy series of treatments. Many follow-up visits are necessary and patient motivation must be high" (Leonardo and Chrisler 1992, 10). With HPV, treatments are directed to infected/abnormal cells. In terms of reoccurrence rates, approximately 25 percent of cervical lesions and/or genital warts return within three months of the first treatment, but this rate can be much higher or lower depending upon the type of HPV and kind of treatment. There are no medical treatments for either the HSV or HPV virus and, therefore, no curative treatments for these infections.

Pain Management

The women discovered that the pain inherent in most treatment options required high levels of motivation and tolerance. The fear of what it would feel like to have their genital tissue frozen, burned, or sliced off had some of the women managing their pain before treatment began. For instance, Haley drew on a memory of comparable pain and imagined how it would feel to have her genital warts frozen with liquid nitrogen:

> I had had plantar warts on my feet before and had those frozen, and so I was thinking about that. I was making that kind of connection and the pain of that, of like having that shot of liquid nitrogen or whatever it is. And they freeze it, and it hurts. I could not walk for two days!

Fears such as this were often, but not always, realized. In general, the women described various degrees of actual pain, depending upon their treatment plan and severity of infection.

Many of the women recalled first having to cope with pain during the evaluative procedures that confirmed the extent/severity of the initial diagnoses. For herpes, cultures of the lesions helped practitioners to recognize how far the infection had spread. Janine described how it felt to have her doctor culture both genital and anal lesions:

> They broke open all of the sores. And I had them anally, and I got them on the outside of the genitals . . . it sounded like he was breaking like 60,000 of them. I'm sure that there weren't that many, but it just took a while. And, he kept apologizing, saying, "I know this is hurting you." But it wasn't so bad as it was like twelve hours later, when I had to go to the bathroom.[3]

For women with cervical HPV, punch biopsies during a colposcopy served a similar function. Some experienced these procedures as sharp pains and cramping. Others, like Amelia, "didn't think it was that bad." She recalled the four punch biopsies of her cervix as "not hurting hardly at all." While women with external HPV rarely underwent biopsies, a few did: Summer described the biopsy of a wart as "very, very, very painful."

The women with external HPV infections (anogenital warts) faced different types of pain, depending upon whether they were treated with liquid nitrogen or trichloroacetic acid applied directly to the warts. Following the biopsy, Summer received liquid nitrogen treatment:

> No one tells you how bad it's gonna' hurt—nobody tells you the kind of pain that you feel . . . I was laying on the table, and they're taking this freezing stuff, and they're placing it on the most sensitive part of your body, and I just felt so sick.

As with many external HPV infections, Summer's warts required several treatments. With the painful memory of this first one, she had to brace herself for repeat treatments that often caused intense pain, without eliminating the warts:

> The treatment was doing nothing: [The warts] weren't shrinking—they weren't going away. By this time, I had more of them. They weren't just in that [initial] area: I had one on the head of my clitoris, I had some inside my labia, and the largest one was still in [my perineum] . . . I couldn't handle it anymore.

Summer's frustration mirrored that of all the women infected with external HPV: None experienced alleviation of symptoms after just one treatment. Many quit Western medical treatment and switched to more holistic approaches of strengthening their immune systems to internally fight the virus. In Summer's case, she stopped using narcotics, reduced her stress, and cut back on smoking cigarettes. Soon after she had made these lifestyle changes she noticed her warts were gone. She admitted, "I don't know what did it—I really don't: Maybe the treatment finally kicked in."

More of the women with external HPV received trichloroacetic acid treatments, where practitioners applied the acid solution directly to the warts, then rinsed it off after a designated amount of time. At the low end of pain, Sierra attested that "it hurt, but not too bad." In fact, she compared it to pain from removal of her plantar wart that, she said, "hurt worse." In contrast Mary, a 51-year-old, white, lower-middle-class professional, remembered that her practitioner had "burned as many [warts] as I could stand because that really is awful." Like Summer, Mary "had to come back in" for repeat treatments, three additional times to have "them all burned off." Monica also remembered the acid treatments "hurting a lot." Natasha, a 20-year-old undergraduate student, mentioned the element of humility as adding to the discomfort of receiving acid treatments: "I was shy, you know, having to get up and spread my legs—[my vagina] seems more like just a body part now than some taboo, sexual body part." Managing shame often overlapped with managing pain.

With internal HPV infections of the cervix, cryosurgery was cited as the most common treatment for mild cases. Haley, who had imagined the pain of her plantar wart removal prior to her cryosurgery, entered her treatment procedure with "that kind of pain envisioned in my head . . . all I could feel was sick." At the sight of the application tool, which looked to her "like a big gun—like a trigger and stuff," Haley began to cry. Her anxiety caused her vaginal muscles to contract to the point that a speculum could not be inserted until a half hour had passed. Then the treatment proved to be "very painful." Louise also remembered it being "incredibly painful":

> I'm like, is there something wrong with me? Because [the practitioners] were like, "Oh, it's not that painful." And I remember thinking I was gonna' pass out after two minutes of being sprayed with [the liquid nitrogen]. And again the pain was just unbelievable the rest of that day.

This case illustrates how pain management was made more difficult when practitioners downplayed the reality that many women experience cryosurgery as severely painful.

In addition to the typical pain from cervical cramping, Amelia experienced the secondary discomfort of a "hot flash" triggered by her cryosurgery. Fortunately, her practitioner had forewarned her that "a very small percentage of women get hot flashes from this." With those words still hanging in the air, Amelia experienced a severe hot flash:

> That was really bad "cause I just didn't know what it was gonna" be like. And [my practitioners] said that my face got redder than anyone that they had ever seen. It was just so uncomfortable. I got really upset because my body was responding in a way that I couldn't control . . . I got very flustered and hot and got kind of choked up, like I was starting to cry.

The physical pain, coupled with embarrassment over not being able to control her body's reaction, left Amelia emotionally and physically drained after cryosurgery.

Those women, with more severe cervical HPV infections, underwent loop electrocautery excision procedures (LEEP), or cone biopsies. As both of these procedures removed large portions of the cervix, the pain was more intense and required a longer time for recovery.

Louise entered a hospital for LEEP, after a practitioner had promised her it would not hurt. In fact, it was only recommended that she "take some Advil." Then she described the procedure as bearable, but the recovery period as "unbelievable—it hurt so bad":

> It felt like somebody was taking a knife and just repetitively stabbing and twisting it in my stomach. I couldn't move: I was just lying in bed. Then I started walking back and forth practically screaming from pain . . . I'm like, "My God, if this [pain] is part of having a kid, I don't want one!"

As she struggled to manage her cervical pain, she also wondered "is there something wrong with me?" She worried that something had gone wrong with her procedure, because her practitioners had told her there "was going to be a little cramping." When a nurse called her the next day to check on her, Louise expressed anger over her pain and confusion over why she had experienced more than cramping. The nurse replied, "Oh, you know why it hurts? Sometimes we cut off your nerve endings and so you have to wait for your nerve endings to die. That must have been what it was." Louise hung up the phone furious that she had not been told about that possibility beforehand.

In contrast to the women with HPV, who had the option of treatments to remove infected tissues, the women living with genital herpes were offered prescriptions for either anti-viral topical creams, or oral medication. These purported to alleviate symptoms, shorten the duration of outbreaks, or possibly stave off an outbreak, when medication was taken at the first pre-outbreak signs, such as tingling in the area, soreness in legs, and other signs one would typically associate with influenza.

These medications did not always work right away. As Tanya explained, her oral medication started to relieve her pain "after maybe the third day, but in the meantime I was getting worse." Her practitioner later recommended that she try taking one pill per day as a preventive measure, and to "experiment with different [medication] schedules" to find out what worked for her body. Diana had been given similar advice by her doctor, taking "sort of a maintenance dose just to make sure that I didn't give [herpes] to [my sexual partner]." However, there are side effects to constantly taking anti-viral medication: "It saps energy . . . the higher doses that you take when you have an outbreak really sap energy." Diana, like several of the other women with herpes, also started taking the amino acid L-lysine, a supplement that has anti-viral properties (Griffith et al. 1987). However, one non-physical side effect of taking herpes medication was its cost. Even Diana, whose salary placed her in the upper-middle-class, commented, "It's expensive."

For reasons of cost and alternative preferences for managing illness, a few of the women with herpes chose not to manage their painful symptoms with medication. Those who sought out health education often learned about the course of this disease. Rhonda, who had contracted herpes in her early 20s, "learned that [outbreaks] usually become less frequent and less severe" over time and chose to not treat her outbreaks, rather to learn the triggers. She commented:

> I don't like taking a lot of medicine, and the cream never did anything for me anyway. So I just kind of let them be, and I know that when I'm really stressed, I'm gonna' get one . . . But, I have noticed it's gotten less frequent, and I do know that sometimes I get them right around my period. Double whammy.

Similarly, Janine did not take medication and noticed that stress triggered her outbreaks. She described managing a recent outbreak, via aspirin and tolerance:

> For the last month, month-and-a-half, I've just been absolutely miserable. I've been to the point of not being able to sleep at night because I'm in so much pain. . . . Aspirin will solve the pains in my legs and in my rear end. It just seems the pain is not necessarily from the lesions.

Pain management in lieu of medication required greater levels of patience.

Cost Management

As evidenced in the above stories, choices to take or not take medication were heavily influenced by cost management. Like Diana's case, practitioners sometimes recommended taking small doses everyday as a preventive measure. Tanya's practitioner had advised her to do this, but living on a graduate student's salary did not allow Tanya to afford "one pill a day—they're pretty expensive." She hopes to be able to begin this type of regimen once she graduates and begins earning a better salary.

Rhonda, diagnosed with herpes at age 18, went to get her prescription filled and found out that 30 pills would cost her $150. She explained her situation: "I was working in a bookstore: I couldn't afford to buy the pills, so I felt completely helpless." Her gynecologist had explained that this medication "was the only way that I was gonna' get better quicker." Constrained by her socioeconomic status, Rhonda had no choice but to manage her symptoms on her own.

Janine faced similar economic barriers from filling a $175 prescription for herpes medication. When she called up her practitioner to express her surprise, and ask for alternative options, she encountered criticism spawned from classism:

> I called him up—I was pissed. And I said, "Why didn't you tell me [about the cost]?" He knew I had lost my job, and he said, "If you'd get yourself a job where you had decent health insurance this wouldn't be a problem." After that, I thought, I will never go back to him again.

This type of incident was typical for women with fewer economic resources, and research has found that the "availability of medical care is still unequally divided along class lines and blame for transmission of diseases is frequently placed on outcast groups" (Leonardo and Chrisler 1992:2). As the above stories detail, treatment for herpes and HPV required enduring physical pain, embarrassment, frustration, and, sometimes, criticism. Consequently, anger became an integral emotional component of the *sexual healing* stage.

Anger Management

Frank (1991) emphasized subjectivity in understanding loss and illness: "The ill person's losses vary according to one's life and illness. We should never question what a person chooses to mourn. One person's losses may seem eccentric to another, but the loss is real enough, and that reality deserves to be honored" (39). STD treatments represented improvement of symptom management, but also highlighted losses as the women found themselves more dependent on the care of medical experts. They had lost the feeling of being in control of their sexual health, and many were angry: With their situation, and with those they held responsible for their infections. This section explores how the women expressed anger over the losses experienced, as they endured painful, costly, and imperfect treatments.

Learning of betrayal often fueled women's feelings of anger during the stage of *sexual healing*. Ingrid, at the time of the interview was still trying to receive HPV treatment having had her practitioner refuse to perform a colposcopy. She expressed anger at her ex-partner, whom she was very certain had infected her:

> Can you believe I dated this human for two-and-a-half years? Can you believe that everybody thought he was so nice and so cool and so wonderful, great, happy, kind, and thoughtful. Asshole, he's an asshole. I hate him—*hate him*. I hope his penis falls off.

Diana remembered feeling similar "rage" when she thought about the man who had betrayed her trust, by knowingly infecting her with HPV, after he had been confronted about infecting a previous partner:

> I really got crazy about it . . . I must admit that I had such rage: This was probably one of the first times ever in my life when I felt like I could go shoot somebody. And I really wanted to shoot his balls off. You know, I didn't really want to kill him. I just wanted to maim him.

It was common for women who had discovered that they were victims of betrayal in the STD anxiety stage to feel anger to the point of wishing bodily harm on their exes.

Summer, who was also dealing with anger over betrayal, described her anger at her ex, in addition to anger at a different kind of loss, that of the ability to feel good about her sexual body. She tied loneliness into her expression of loss and anger:

> It was something so intimate and so beautiful turned into something so painful and so ugly, and made me feel so empty, you know. And [my practitioner] walked out of the room, and I'm laying there with my legs together just bawling because there was nobody there, especially the asshole who did it. There was just nobody there.

Summer, and other women who were single at the time of treatment, feared going through this process alone and were often angry as a result. However, women who had sexual partners at the time of treatment also felt fear and anger, though their focus shifted to how the success or failure of their treatments would impact their partners. Francine shared this point of view:

> The feelings were fear and anger: I was really angry that the person who I thought gave it to me had been so dishonest. I was angry with him anyway because of all the dishonesty. I was even angrier now that he would bring this into my marriage . . . I was certainly concerned about my own health and real concerned that I would pass it on to my husband.

Her example shows how anger at betrayal combined with fear of harming loved ones, and fear for her own health increased the difficulty of managing her emotions during treatments.

In the few cases where the persons responsible for transmission tried to ease the women's treatment burdens, anger still surfaced. Janine admitted, "I was angry, and I shouldn't have been angry with him . . . he was very upset that I got it, and he immediately went and got a culture and blood test, and he knew he had it." She recalled how her ex-partner had offered to help pay for her medication, but she still felt that he was "not doing enough." She owned up to feeling irrational: "I don't know what I wanted—I was angry."

The two women who had contracted STDs as a result of sexual assaults expressed additional dimensions of anger. Monica, who had survived a date rape attempt without "officially" losing her virginity, mourned the fact that she had not even enjoyed sexual pleasures before contracting external HPV:

> I hadn't even gotten to enjoy my sexual life, and it was already taken away from me. I was really angry, actually . . . looking at all the people that were so irresponsible: Hearing about my friends that weren't using condoms and having sex with these people, having sex with their boyfriends because their boyfriends convinced them that it's okay to have sex without a condom. And I'm the only one out of all my friends that doesn't even have sex, made the decision not to do this, and it's me that gets this.

Overall, Monica felt that her condition was "unfair" and the treatment process brought out more anger of this perceived injustice. Molly, who had contracted cervical HPV from a rapist, expressed how the fact that a sexual assault was the cause of her having to receive treatments added to her pain and anger: "Since the source is the rapist, I have this extra feeling to carry around with me, you know, thinking that is like another dimension of the hurt, of the violation, of the wrong."

Constructing the Meaning of "Chronic"

In addition to negotiating relationships with practitioners and managing difficult aspects of treatment, the women also had to come to terms with the incurable nature of their infections, in order to cognitively grasp the meaning of healing. They discovered that chronic illness not only meant that their infections were "officially" incurable, but also that the treatment process could take from one month to six years to achieve desired alleviation of symptoms. In addition, the women faced the prospect that their viral infections could lay dormant and reemerge as symptomatic later on in their lives, during periods of high stress and/or hormonal change.

In cases when practitioners presented inaccuracies during diagnosis and treatment, the incurable nature of these STDs took longer to inform the women's illness definitions. For Molly, her practitioner did not introduce the fact that HPV was chronic until after her cone biopsy procedure at a follow-up exam:

Another thing that emerged this go around was he said, "It's not that uncommon for it to come back. This is sort of what we expect." And I remember thinking that I hadn't known that I should expect it to come back. Like we'll do this cone surgery, and then it'll be over [except for follow-up] Pap smears. But I wasn't aware that [HPV] was an ongoing issue that I would live with . . . Now I have this feeling that I need to know a whole lot more because it's something I'm gonna' live with.

Those women who required repeat treatments to eliminate HPV infections expressed how it was finding out that they required another treatment that made them recognize their illness statuses as chronic. Pam, who had been initially diagnosed with a cervical HPV infection and received cryosurgery, later was diagnosed with genital warts: "They were on the labia and inside lip—this made me feel more contagious." Helena, 31 years old and hoping to marry someday, echoed the emotional strain of feeling that her body was still infected and contagious: "When the warts came back, that's when it really, totally hit me that, okay, yeah, I'm like dirty for life."

After having had cryosurgery, Haley received normal Pap smear results and felt that her HPV was behind her, but the news of her next Pap smear showing abnormal cells, "really freaked me out":

I was like, "Oh, no—I already have some fraction of my cervix pretty much gone. I really don't want to go through this again." And, at that point, I was a freshman in college and was just thinking more in terms of my future, not being able to have children and things like that. And, like if I had to go through this again, like how many times can they do cryo? How many times until [HPV] is gonna' take over my entire cervix? What's the extent of this really gonna' be?

Haley asked these questions of her practitioner who explained, "The thing about this disease is that it's so unpredictable." She remembered her practitioner saying, "Even if you do the cryo [sic], and we get what's there, it can come back, or maybe it never will."

Haley was not alone in her fears that the chronic nature of these infections could cause problems for future fertility. Francine had first contracted genital warts that had never returned after an initial treatment. However, her herpes infection proved far less easy to manage and left her afraid for her future:

> Since it was viral, [herpes] would be life-long . . . the stories I had heard about herpes were much more horror stories of people not being able to have sex very much again their whole life. And, here I'd just entered into this relatively new relationship with somebody, and we were really happy. And, I was just so bummed. So, I thought that herpes meant infertility—it concerned me because I already knew that it could affect the whole birth process, and we had talked about having a baby someday. I didn't know if that was jeopardized.

For Francine, and other women who eventually wanted to have children, this issue became the most feared aspect of having a chronic STD.

Cancer arose as an equally prevalent and sometimes connected long-term fear for those with cervical HPV infections. In describing how she felt after being treated for genital warts, Monica summarized:

> The scariest thing for me is [the issue of having] children—it's the most important thing in my life . . . I know [about] the whole cervical cancer thing . . . I think that's the scariest part for me, in the long-term what it can do to my reproductive system.

Sandy, 21 years old at the time of the interview, expressed similar concerns and wanted to find out how HPV had been "linked to cancer." Natasha, initially diagnosed and treated for external warts, remained concerned "about the internal [warts] a lot too because I had some burning during sex the other day, and I like kind of freaked out and went to the doctor to see if there's anything wrong." At the time of the interview she was waiting for these Pap smear results and feeling "more concerned about cervical cancer."

Several of the women described how, after successful treatments, they found it easy to lapse into forgetting that their infections were chronic. Monica remarked, "Unfortunately, when you don't have symptoms everyday, and when it's not something you have to face everyday illness-wise, it's very easy to forget about." Likewise, a couple of months had passed between Ashley's colposcopy and cryosurgery, and she confessed, "I guess I hadn't really thought about what I had 'cause [there had been] such a long waiting period in between." However, the issue of permanence regains poignancy during each gynecological exam that has followed the conclusion of her treatment:

> It's like every time I go, when I have a gynecology appointment, it's just like I get it all back again. Like I'm diseased and dirty, like it just reminds me all over again. [This past time] I put my legs up in the stirrups, and it was horrible. I cried—felt the whole thing, like everything came back, everything.

Feelings of being permanently *damaged goods* strengthened during treatments and follow-up exams.

In order to pursue healing and recovery, the women had to negotiate relationships with practitioners, manage physical, financial, and emotional strains, and reconcile the meaning of having a chronic illness. I began this chapter with Frank's (1991) question about how one finds value in experiencing an illness from which one cannot fully recover. He found, "The answer seems to be focusing less on recovery and more on renewal" (Frank 1991, 2). In the next chapter, and final stage in the process of how incurable STDs transform women's sexual selves, I explore the issue of renewal.

7 Reintegrating the Sexual Self

All of the women experienced elements of the previous five stages. Having been diagnosed and treated for incurable STDs, they (1) reexamined myths of STD invincibility, (2) faced anxieties over their transforming sexual health statuses, (3) became stigmatized patients by virtue of diagnoses, (4) struggled to individually manage their stigma, and (5) endured the multifaceted duress of medical treatments. Their final challenge was to incorporate new sexual attitudes and behaviors into how they saw themselves as sexual beings. Sexual-self *reintegration* entailed finding a balance between risk awareness and the desire for romantic intimacy. They could not return to the "ignorance is bliss" mentality of *sexual invincibility*, and they had to come to terms with the higher levels of anxiety, shame, and stigma that had permeated earlier portions of their illness experiences.

The six stages of sexual-self transformation described in this book embody Mechanic's (1982) view of how individuals behave throughout the trajectory of an illness: "Illness behavior is a dynamic process through which the person defines the problems, struggles with them, and attempts to achieve a comfortable accommodation" (19). The majority, but not all, of the women I studied had entered this final stage of trying to achieve "comfortable accommodation" by the time of our interviews. In the *reintegration* stage, the women reached a point where they felt that they had reclaimed their sexual selves from illness. This final chapter of their stories reflects Frank's (1998) finding: "This reclaiming is not a sudden epiphany but a slow, gradual process" (204). For this reason, those women who had only recently been diagnosed and treated prior to being interviewed had not yet entered this stage.

Incomplete Reintegration

A few of the women who had been living with herpes and/or HPV for several years ceased sexual-self transformation at earlier stages: These women had undergone treatments, yet remained focused on feeling contagious and worried about stigma management. They did the best that they could do with the resources at hand because, while "illness can lead us to live differently, accepting it is neither easy nor self-evident" (Frank 1991, 3).

As mentioned in Chapter 5, celibacy was one strategy employed to delay the discomfort of disclosure. While the majority of the women who initially employed this strategy eventually decided to disclose in order to facilitate new romantic relationships, both Mary and Marissa did not. Mary, who had contracted HPV in her 40s while single, opted for long-term celibacy once she entered the *immoral patient* stage. Her practitioner had explained that her cervical and external HPV infections were sexually transmitted and contagious. Mary remembered feeling, "so humiliated," and admitted: "I have not had sex since. Not that anybody would have sex with me, but I still would *never, ever*." Part of her reasoning was that she had learned that standard "male" condoms (those that encase the penis) did not provide enough protection from the skin-to-skin contact that transmits genital warts. Instead, she was told to use the "big [condom] that covers the lips of your vagina"; by this she was referring to the "female" condom.[1] While Mary's treatments proved successful in that she never experienced additional outbreaks, her practitioner's warning that HPV "could come back" led her to "quit thinking about sex . . . it's completely out of my life."

Marissa, 31-years-old at the time of our interview, expressed similar emotions, stating that cervical and external HPV infections had "really messed me up." She related a recent story about her trip to London where she had met a "cute Irish guy." She remembered him "hitting on" her and "trying his damnedest" to talk her into having sex. At this point, fears of contracting HIV dominated Marissa's thoughts: "All I had heard was you gotta' be careful because AIDS is like rampant in London." Then, she thought, "Well, I have this other issue, and I just don't want to give [HPV] to somebody." While her sexual health fears over a potential one-night-stand were well founded, Marissa expressed distress that she has since avoided all sexual situations with men. During our interview that occurred six years after her diagnosis and treatment, Marissa summarized, "I still feel like I don't know where I stand with [HPV]." She felt "too afraid" to risk having a sexual relationship.

While Mary, Marissa, Hillary, and Julia were the only ones to have chosen long-term celibacy, many of the women expressed desires to "escape" the challenges of reintegration by returning to celibacy. Gloria, a single-mother with two children at home, had struggled with sexual relationships, often facing rejection after disclosing her STD status to partners. Having recently had a relationship end just prior to our interview, she asserted:

> I'm starting to feel like maybe I don't need a man in my life . . .
> Maybe I don't want men in my life because it's so frustrating to
> have to go through this: Telling people. It's humiliating and
> embarrassing. It's so frustrating to have to think about the idea
> that I can give somebody else fucking herpes, that I don't need
> this shit.

However, her anger changed into tentative hope when she admitted, "At the same time, I'm lonely." She concluded, "Maybe I'll just lay off men for a while," and talked about wanting to eventually find a man with whom she could have a loving, open, and healthy relationship. Gloria's struggle to find a balance between the stigmatizing nature of her infections and her desire for intimacy was the most common outcome, one that motivated almost all of the women to reconstruct the meanings of sexual health issues and revise their approaches to romantic relationships. Transforming these two aspects of their sexual lives resulted in them finally being able to experience a reintegrated sexual self.

Redefining Sexual Health Issues

In order to "reclaim" their sexual selves from illness, the women had to redefine the meanings of sexual health issues. Reintegration required the women to focus inward and incorporate their STD illness experiences into their sexual health attitudes, sexual health behaviors, and gender roles.

Sexual Health Attitudes

The women viewed their changed attitudes about sexual health as key parts of their new sexual selves. One way this occurred was by reframing their chronic STD experience as a "wake-up call" that alerted them to the reality of sexual health risks. Another aspect of attitudinal change was increased expectations of sexual partners' sexual health practices. Finally, some of the women experienced an attitudinal shift in reference to sexual health practitioner interactions.

Many of the women put a positive label on their experiences with chronic STDs by viewing their illness experiences as catalysts for taking a new and better stance that sexual health was both precarious and precious. Chris, who had come to terms with her herpes infection as a single person and was still interested in dating, expressed that she saw contracting "HIV or HPV" from a future partner as a possibility and credited her past experiences for her new attitude. Similarly, Diana, who was single and dated into her early 40s, viewed contracting herpes and genital warts as "the AIDS wakeup call." Ingrid, who contracted HPV from her first college boyfriend, also believed that contracting this STD had made her "more aware" because she realized that she "could have gotten a worse" STD. Sierra, who worked for a sexual health clinic where she learned about the range of sexually transmitted diseases, explained that she reframed having HPV as a benefit because it changed her sexual health attitudes before she contracted a "more severe" disease: "I don't have AIDS, I can deal with that . . . [HPV] is not as serious as having HIV or AIDS."

Their new sexual health attitudes also included revised expectations of sexual partners. As disclosure had become a key part of dating, attitudes about rejection changed to reflect the women's newfound belief that sexual health took priority over ego. For example, Haley, in her early 20s and dating at the time of our interview, explained that she now expected a partner to tell her about his STD status and accept her disclosure. If a man were to reject her on the basis of her disclosure, she said she would take the following position:

> It would just mean that he was pretty shallow anyway. And that if he was serious about me, and if he were serious about developing any type of close relationship, then he would accept that about me. And he wouldn't think less of me . . . if he did, then he wasn't serious about it in the first place, and he'd probably have some issues of his own. So I wouldn't take [his rejection] to heart.

Haley's new attitude reflected knowledge that avoiding STD risk also meant avoiding certain types of partners.

Ingrid also felt that HPV had changed her attitude about sexual relationships. Her illness experiences left her with a habit of assuming partners had sexual experiences that had put them at risk for contracting STDs. She imagined her beliefs would translate into going on a date and then getting "tested" for STDs before sexual contact:

> I'm gonna' assume that he has a sexual history, and I just don't want to be lied to again. I also don't want someone to do what I did: Give [an STD] to someone without knowing you have it. And so I feel like if it can be addressed in a way like, "Let's go in together [for testing]. Oh this will be so fun: If you have an STD, you can tell me, it's okay."

While her humorous telling of this scenario was clearly tongue-in-cheek, Ingrid's general sentiment was one of promoting honesty and awareness of sexual health over conforming to typical dating norms.

The final way in which the women's sexual health attitudes changed was with regard to practitioner interactions. This type of attitudinal shift was found among women who had encountered practitioners with poor bedside manner, lacking educational skills, and preferences to exclude patients from deciding treatment options. Lola, who had received treatment from a doctor who became defensive when she had asked him about her Internet research on HPV, described how her sexual self had grown to include the role of being her own medical educator and advocate:

> Whatever may be wrong with me, for whatever future diagnostic purposes, the first thing I'm gonna' do is go and do my own research because I don't feel like I can fully trust what the doctor is telling me. And it's not something necessarily that [doctors] do deliberately. A lot of times I think that doctors just get in this 'doctor mode.' They see and deal with this stuff every day, so that there's a certain desensitization that they go through.

By the time Lola had reached the reintegration stage, her anger towards her practitioner had decreased substantially; she was able to see the flaws in the system of care, rather than just focusing on the individual practitioner. She went on to detail the tangible benefits to being a self-educated patient:

> [Practitioners] might ask you, like my doctor did, "Do you have any questions?" But, you don't even know what questions to ask . . . when I have future medical problems, I'm gonna' go out and do my own research so that I can learn more, get a better hold on what [my condition] is, how it happened, and what's involved with treating it so that I can have the questions.

Lola, embracing new attitudes about sexual health practitioner interactions had become proactive in her search to figure out why her past encounters had been disappointing and how future ones might be improved. Her story was representative of the majority of women who had had unsatisfactory practitioner interactions and developed a 'take charge' stance towards sexual health education.

Sexual Health Behaviors

While attitudinal changes transformed certain aspects of how the women saw themselves as sexual beings, commitments to behavioral changes strengthened their resolve to maintain their new sexual selves. Health researchers (Leonardo and Chrisler 1992, 10) have noted the necessity of behavioral changes for individuals living with chronic STDs:

> The instruction to abstain from sex or use a condom . . . is not as serious a problem for diseases such as gonorrhea and Chlamydia, which can be cured in a few weeks, as it is for diseases such as venereal warts . . . Changes in sexual behavior must be life long for those diagnosed with herpes or AIDS.

The women came to see themselves as individuals who acted with a newfound awareness in matters of sexual health: Including sexual interactions, non-sexual interactions, and private interactions with themselves.

Sexual interactions required revised sexual health behaviors to achieve the new goals of preventing re-infection or new infections. In addition to adjusting how they had sexual relations, an issue expanded on later in this chapter, the women also adopted new standards for STD testing and reciprocity of disclosure.

Several of the women shared examples of how they had become advocates for sexual health testing when a potential partner had historically ignored his/her sexual health. Summer, whose genital warts had not recurred since she had strengthened her immune system, related a recent "pre-sex" discussion with a partner:

> We sat there, and we just talked. He asked me about all kinds of STDs: Things he didn't know about, things he felt uncomfortable about, and that he had been with this girl for a while and she had cheated on him. He [still] hadn't been tested—he never had been tested for certain things. I said, "Go get an STD screening. It doesn't hurt you. If anything, it makes you feel more at ease."

In Haley's case, her current boyfriend had not been tested since his prior sexual relationship had ended. She used humor to express her strong feelings about STD testing when she told him, "I'm gonna' drag you by the arm to the doctor and go in there with you." Diana also adopted an assertive approach; however, having already contracted herpes and HPV, she focused on protecting herself against HIV. She role-played her new approach to interacting with potential sexual partners: "After this incident [of contracting herpes], I started asking guys about HIV: 'Have you had an HIV test? Do you have the results? When was the last time?'" All three of these women had revised their stances on STD testing to reflect the belief that their bodies and sexual selves deserved protection.

Other women described new ideas of how they should act in matters of testing, disclosure, and communication among sexual partners. For example, Sarah, who had not had a recurrence of HPV for four years, explained her new approach to protecting her sexual health: "It comes down to being honest with your partner, getting yourself examined, getting them examined, and then deciding in an educated way what risks you are going to take." She acknowledged the fact that having a goal to avoid infection entailed learning about risks and negotiating with sexual partners. She had discovered that to find a balance between sexual health goals and the realities of medical and human imperfections meant acting with an awareness that there were no guarantees when living with an incurable STD. Chris also favored mutual disclosure, after both she and a prospective partner were tested: "My ideal scenario would be I'd meet someone and you know things were progressing in that direction, and I could open things up [about my STD status], and then he would be frank with me, too." She summarized, "It's preferable for me to be fairly outspoken about it." Women like those above hoped to set "good examples" for their partners by changing their behaviors with regard to testing, disclosure, and honest communication about sexual health matters.

A few of the women mentioned having made health behavior changes that did not involve sexual contexts. For example, Monica, who had contracted genital warts from an attempted date rape, described how she had turned taking showers into a sexual health self-exam: "It's a habit: I'll check [for new genital warts] when I'm showering and washing—I'll check more carefully now than I usually would before [having been diagnosed]." Sarah, who had been treated for HPV over five years before being interviewed, also described checking for warts but used a mirror. However she noted that the longer it had been since her last outbreak, the less frequently she felt the need to examine herself.

A few of the women with herpes mentioned another behavioral change. They had become vigilant about preventing the possibility of non-sexual transmissions. As herpes lesions can manifest as fluid-filled blisters, some women had learned about the possibility for contamination of surfaces (such as toilet seats) and materials (such as washcloths).[2] Janine, for instance, kept track of which bath towel she used when her grown children came to visit: "When the kids are here, I take my towel out of the bathroom, and I really try to be careful." Whether the behavioral changes were of a sexual nature or not, the women had come to be cautious about matters of sexual health.

Sexual Gender Norms and Roles

In this chapter, I have described how the women transformed their approaches to romantic relationships and integrated new sexual health attitudes and behaviors to reformulate their sexual selves. These aspects of reintegration brought relief from feeling victimized by their illnesses because the women experienced their new sexual selves as being assertive, self-sufficient, intelligent, and self-protective—all traits that railed against traditional feminine gender norms of passivity, dependency, naiveté, and other-directedness. In order to experience their reintegrated sexual selves, the women had to challenge and systematically shun much of what they had been socialized to believe about the role of women in heterosexual relationships. Those who had self-identified as bisexual or lesbian described having had to put less energy into this aspect of reintegration. However, the remaining thirty-seven heterosexual women found the task difficult but worth their efforts.

Leonardo and Chrisler (1992) noted that many of the behavioral changes that could help a woman protect her health also put her in the position of being a gender deviant. For example, they found that "women who do not feel that they can exercise control in their relationships cannot initiate the required changes" (Leonardo and Chrisler 1992:10). Similarly, "If a woman begins to ask a man about his sexual history, it may appear that she is trying to question his authority and cause conflict . . . women have been socialized to put the needs and desires of others before their own" (Leonardo and Chrisler 1992, 7–8). The feminine stance of other-directedness makes it difficult for a woman to obtain vital information about her partner's health. These researchers also addressed commitment to condom usage: "Condom use, like talking to one's partner about STDs, is dependent on a woman's ability to be assertive in an intimate relationship. Traditional gender roles require women to follow the lead of their partners in romantic and sexual situations." (Leonardo and Chrisler 1992, 8) For all of these reasons, the women in my study who reached the stage of *reintegration* explained how they had adopted new gender norms and roles as part of piecing together new sexual selves.

Assertiveness versus Passivity

The women described switching from being passive to being assertive about sexual health issues in relationships as an important new gender norm. For instance, Ashley, in her early 20s and hoping to get married someday, discussed this when she stated how her experiences with HPV had changed her formerly feminine approach towards handling disclosure in a romantic relationship. She asserted, "I would approach it much differently than I would have before: Like instead of being all passive [and saying something] like, 'Are you gonna' break up with me?'" Rather, Ashley contended she would say and feel the following:

> Probably before we got any further than kissing, I would let him know right away [that I have HPV]. Like there's no doubt about it . . . I'm gonna' be like, "This is what I have. If you aren't okay with this, oh, well." And truly, that's the way it is. I mean if someone has a problem with [me having HPV], then that's not someone I want in my life.

She believed that having survived the stresses and strains of living with HPV had "definitely" made her a more assertive sexual being. Likewise, Natasha felt more assertive as a result of managing genital warts: "I found myself saying 'No' to people that I wouldn't have said 'No' to in the past." Looking back on her pre-STD self, she realized that she had been both passive and dependent on others for her self-esteem: "I had a problem of finding confidence in myself and expressing how I feel."

Self-sufficiency versus Dependency

The women also explained how they had started playing a more self-sufficient role in sexual relationships and relying less on their partners for affirmation. Chris, for example, remembered her pre-herpes sexual self as having needed the praise of men to feel attractive and desirable, even when this dependency required her to ignore her own feelings. She recalled one of her early relationships in which she had noticed a suspicious sore on her boyfriend's penis, but decided to consent to sexual relations: "Ten years ago, I didn't want to *not* have sex with [a boyfriend] because the relationship was so important to my ego." Coming from a place of dependency, Chris' need for affirmation outweighed her gut instincts that this was not a healthy decision. In contrast, she now argued that gendered "power issues" would have to change such that "women wouldn't be in the position of seeing [a suspicious sore] on somebody's penis and going along with it." From her new vantage point, she believed she had the self-sufficiency to make tough choices, if need be, in sexual situations.

Summer provided another example of the shift away from a reliance on sexual partners for sexual validation. As a bisexual, she had had both male and female sexual partners to whom she had looked for affirmation. She described her pre-HPV sexual self: "I was at a point where [my sexual health] didn't matter to me. I felt like, 'You want my body, fine. As long as it just makes me feel better." Reflecting back on her past, she commented, "It's really sad that I was there, but I'm better now." Summer credited her sexual-self transformation to having contracted an incurable STD: "I feel that if I hadn't gotten the HPV, I would have never changed that lifestyle." As I mentioned earlier, Summer had become devout about protecting her sexual health: "I will never have sex again without a condom . . . period. That's just the way it is." Her strong tone and word choice represented a new strength she now embodied.

Intelligence versus Naiveté

Several of the women elaborated on another aspect of revised gender roles: Having "played dumb" in pre-STD sexual interactions so that male partners would be drawn to their feminine sexual naiveté. Sam, 34 years old at the time of the interview, expressed disgust with how she had behaved in the past, describing her observations of women downplaying their intelligence when it came to sexual health decisions: "Women have awareness about how to [protect themselves], but don't insist on condoms, even though they know the risk." After admitting to me that she had often acted this way, Sam grew angry: "It just doesn't make sense, especially not for smart, confident women—why is it that confident, capable women, who know what they're supposed to do, don't do it?" Her experiences with HPV had helped her to be proud of her sexual health knowledge and to deviate from a norm she had grown to hate.

Self-protective versus Other-directed Attitudes

Finally, women noted that having been other-directed in past sexual relationships had led them to make decisions that endangered their sexual health. For instance, Louise, who had held "very liberal" attitudes about sex as an undergraduate, remembered how this attitude had lead to her risking pregnancy and STDs with a male partner in college: "He entered me without a condom, and that was something that I was really not psyched about." She attributed allowing unprotected intercourse to having had concerns for his feelings: "I think I've always felt guilt for insisting on condoms because, almost uniformly, every guy's complained." At the time of our interview, Louise insisted that her health and well-being had become her top priorities. Sierra bluntly expressed having held a similar belief that men's sexual needs took precedence in heterosexual relationships: "Sometimes in a relationship I felt like it was just a requirement that you have sex with your partner . . . I still was so into pleasing other people that I just did what was good for them." Sierra shared Louise's current belief that putting her own needs first was the only way in which she could protect her sexual health from further damage.

Reinventing Romantic Relationships

In order to redefine sexual health issues, the women had faced the challenge of revising relevant attitudes and behaviors, which in turn motivated reformulations of their gender norms and roles. Romantic relationships then proved to be the primary type of setting in which the women's sexual selves were tested. Weitz (1991, 102) noted similar phenomena in individuals living with HIV: "In addition to devastating one's body, HIV disease can also devastate one's social life . . . some relationships end and others become strained." This type of strain shaped the women's choices to date and reenter the world of sexual relationships.

Researchers on STDs among African women found that they "identified more interpersonal issues, such as the effect of infection on trust in the relationship," as their lasting concern (Pitts et al. 1995, 1302). The women I interviewed also identified the issue of trust within romantic relationships as a focus during this stage. For this reason, dating took on different levels of meaning, in terms of who they were as sexual beings and their expectations of sexual partners. Reinventing romantic relationships challenged the women to revise dating practices to include disclosure, to create new "safer" means of having sex, to overcome feelings of guilt, and to develop new approaches to pregnancy and childbirth.

Disclosure

While a few of the women made the choice to only date men who were similarly infected, the majority came to view disclosure of their STD statuses as an integral part of dating. In Chapter 5, I discussed preventive and cathartic disclosures as stigma management strategies employed immediately following diagnosis. Preventive disclosures transformed into practiced, routine interactions for the single women, who continued to date after receiving treatments. These women developed strategies for telling partners and for coping with their partners' reactions.

Each of the women who dated had an opinion on the optimal timing of when to reveal their STD status. In an unusual case, Chris was able to disclose prior to having met her potential date: She answered a personal ad and disclosed in her phone message when she said, "This is really premature, but you should know that I have herpes, and I know this may stop you from calling me back, but you should know up front." She admitted, "You know, I'm still kinda' struggling with that disclosure." However, she felt it was easier to disclose to this total stranger. She explained, "I have no investment in making this guy like me at all: It's really fifty-fifty. If he calls me, that's great. If he doesn't, hey, so what." Chris had not heard back from this man at the time of our interview, which took place only days after she had left this message. At this point, she felt that this type of "pre-emptive" disclosure was easier than "if I see somebody in a bar and my little heart's pounding."

Several of the women preferred to broach the subject of STDs once it became clear that there was mutual sexual interest, but prior to any sexual situation that could risk transmission. For example, Louise shared that disclosure "would never be at the last minute, but sort of if it looked like we were really interested in each other." Diana also chose to bring up her STD status before her current relationship became sexual:

> I brought it up before we had sex. I think he wanted to have sex, and I said, "Look, there're some things I think we need to talk about." And I was agonizing, you know, weeks and weeks and weeks before trying to figure out how I was gonna' tell him, and trying to get help on how to tell him. I had some friends who said, "Oh, don't tell him." And I'm like, "No, I can't do that."

The women who made decisions to disclose early in relationships often shared Diana's sentiment of it being the "right" thing to do. In Diana's case, she had been betrayed and did not want to wrong another person in this way.

Other women put off disclosing until sexual contact appeared to be imminent. Janine, who had only dated men from a herpes support group since being diagnosed, had recently started dating a man without herpes. She felt insecure about disclosing and tried to avoid it until "we were kind of like making out, and I could tell he wanted it to go farther." Gloria also preferred to "wait to tell men" and outlined her reasons:

> One, is it worth telling them? In other words, am I interested in having sex with this man? Secondly, [I'd wait] to let them get to know me a little bit more, to find out whether or not I am someone that they want to take a chance with. Because it's possible they may not want to, and that's fine. But at least by telling them, and giving them an opportunity to get to know me, then they can make a conscious choice.

Gloria also admitted that her timing of disclosure was dependent upon "how pushy they are [to have sex] . . . if they're real pushy, then you tell them right away and get rid of them." She illustrated a possible benefit to disclosure as a device to "scare off" the "pushy" and otherwise undesirable men.

Still a few of the women held off on disclosure until after they had already been sexually intimate with partners. This subgroup did not make these decisions lightly, but often acted out of a strong fear of rejection. For example, Monica believed it was better to hold off disclosure, even if a relationship became sexual, until she felt that the relationship was "stable." She feared that telling a partner too quickly could have negative consequences, not only to the relationship, but also to her sexual self: "It's so easy for [my partner] just to hear that I have [an STD] and be like, 'No way!' You know, that would just take your whole sexuality away from you with that one little sentence . . . that's definitely scary to me."

Rhonda's story highlighted other aspects of this dilemma. About a month into her first serious relationship after having received a herpes diagnosis, Rhonda remembered, "I had a very big crisis because I realized I had to tell [my boyfriend]." The idea of disclosure "was really scary" because she saw her relationship as being "at a point where it wasn't serious enough, where there was no real commitment, and I felt like he wouldn't feel like it was something worth sticking with. . . . I was very scared that I was gonna' tell him, and he was gonna' run." Ultimately her "responsibility to be honest with him" grew greater than her fears, and she disclosed after they had "had sex maybe a couple of times."

In addition to timing, the content and style of disclosures varied greatly. Women who had less practice often stumbled into revealing the truth. Janine had put off disclosing until her date had made it clear that he wanted to have sex:

> I just go, "We're not having sex." And he goes, "Is there a reason why?" And I said, "No. We're just not having sex. I haven't known you long enough." And he goes, "I understand." Then, I think he was wondering, because I'd also told him I'd like to do my [dissertation] research on [STDs]. So he goes, "But is there a reason?" And I said, "Well yes, but I really hadn't planned to tell you like this. I hadn't planned to tell you now."

In contrast, some of the women used educational approaches to disclose. For instance, Louise shared her typical spiel that included statistics:

> I should probably let you know that I had surgery a year ago for a virus called HPV . . . They estimate that 62 percent of people have it, but they just don't know it. It's easier to transmit male to female than female to male, but I just wanted to put that out there . . . it's the same virus that gives genital warts.

Ingrid, a sexual health peer educator, also drew on educational resources to assist with disclosure. She "pulled out the handy sexual health 'everything-you-need-to-know' notebook," points to the page on HPV and said, "I have this." They then discussed prevalence statistics, modes of transmission, and ways to have safer sex.

The women's (potential) sexual partners' reactions were as varied as the disclosure strategies. Louise, who favored disclosing early via an educational approach, found that her partners "would inspect their penis for the next week or two" and often told her, "Thanks for telling me." For her, this pattern of disclosure interactions "wasn't a big deal." Similarly, Ingrid's educational stance and early timing created a comfortable atmosphere in which her partner asked questions and expressed concern for her health. The statistics she had shared with him made an impression, as he responded by saying, "I don't think you're gross at all. I mean shit, 80 percent of the population has it: I probably have it." Their disclosure interaction had a positive effect on Ingrid's view of her sexual self and of their relationship: "[HPV] had definitely been sort of a blow to my ego, but [his reaction to my disclosure] made me trust him about ten trillion times more."

Post-disclosure reaction proved to be more tenuous for women who had not included education components within their disclosures. For example, Janine, who had disclosed when a sexual encounter felt imminent, faced a partner whose initial understanding response to her not wanting to have sex switched to confusion and fear of contracting herpes:

> I told him, and he kind of backed off really fast. He goes, "Oh, what do you mean? Like now's not a safe time?" And I said,

"No, actually now is probably a safe time, but we're not having sex." And he said, "Oh, okay, fine." And we're going out this week, so it was a really positive experience. I really didn't know how it would go.

Janine's partner had made the erroneous assumption that she would only have told him if she was having an outbreak, i.e.,if it was "not a safe time." While she viewed this experience as "positive," it remained to be seen how he would respond to learning about the risks of transmission during latent phases of the virus. Similarly, Diana's partner appreciated that she had disclosed prior to having sexual intercourse, but responded with fear of contagion:

> But then he didn't want to touch me anywhere near my genitals . . . [disclosure] has probably been—aside from the actual incident [of contracting herpes]—the most painful part. That is meeting somebody who's really nice and who really is turned off by the idea.

Diana's story underscored the fact that timing was not enough to insure a positive response from a partner.

However, the women who delayed disclosures until after sexual contact were more likely to report negative reactions from partners. Rhonda, who had put off disclosure until after sex, found that her partner "was very taken aback." She recalled that he had reacted to her disclosure by saying, "I wish you had told me before." Haley had also delayed disclosure until after she and her partner had become sexually intimate; however, she had oral sex and disclosed when he began to "push" for intercourse. Her partner responded with anger: "Every time I've gone down on you, I could have gotten something on my mouth?" Even though she tried to explain to him that the risks were low for oral transmission from a treated cervical infection, he refused to spend the night, and Haley "just felt dirty." Negative outcomes from disclosing to partners forced some of the women to temporarily refocus on stigma management as these interactions tested their reintegrated sexual selves.

Sexual Intimacy

Once the women had gotten past disclosure, they faced the challenge of adjusting the ways in which they had sexual intercourse. Some of the women perfected the art of foreplay and avoided physical contact that could transmit their viruses. Ashley explained that she and her partner "would do everything except sex—we were fooling around, but no sex." If "fooling around" included oral sex, the women who had learned that their STDs could be transmitted orally also adjusted these behaviors. Sierra has developed a routine for oral sex:

> We kind of like check each other out, you know, and look for stuff. And I've looked on him. But I don't think it's so much that I'm so worried. Like I think we're so open about it that it's like, "Oh, let me see how you're looking." You know, "Have you found anything? Is anything there? No. Okay."

While Sierra's example illustrates how oral sex could remain positive in the light of new sexual health protocol, Ashley and Diana both experienced difficulties having "safer" oral sex. Ashley stated, "I have a really hard time enjoying oral sex now." She remained "really uncomfortable" about her partner performing oral sex on her because of the possible risks to his health. Diana went so far as to say, "Oral sex is definitely off limits since I have herpes." Neither she nor her partner wanted to risk him becoming infected.

Only a few of the women had been educated about the risks of transmitting HPV and herpes via manual contact. Those who had access to this information had learned that if a partner touched skin (oral or genital) that was infected and actively "shedding" the virus and then that partner touched their own or their partner's uninfected skin, transmission could occur. Sarah explained how she and her boyfriend had both been treated for HPV and adjusted their manual stimulation behaviors:

> I wasn't sure like if [our HPV infections] were gonna' come back or what was going on. Literally, when I was with my boyfriend, I washed my hands and then would touch him. I would not touch myself and he would not touch himself, if we were

touching each other, because we both had the virus, and we're trying to like stay safe.

The above examples highlighted how chronic STD infection motivated changes in how the women sexually interacted with partners, even when penetrative intercourse was not an issue.

However, most of the women wanted to continue to have penetrative intercourse with partners and, therefore, mastered consistent and correct use of latex condoms as a way to reduce the risks of transmission. Diana and her whose partner, who had initially been afraid to touch her immediately following disclosure, "tried to do as well as we could with using condoms and trying to make sure that there's no way in which [herpes and HPV] might infect him." The women commonly developed very strong behavioral stances on condom usage. Haley asserted: "We always used condoms. I was on the pill still and I made him wear a condom all the time. I didn't even let him touch me with his penis at all unless he had a condom on. I mean I was really adamant about it." Many of the women believed that condoms were a sexual necessity.

Religious terminology was common among women who took this strong stance on condom usage. For Sierra, her genital warts infection inspired her to change her method of birth control: "Since then I've gone off the pill . . . so we use condoms religiously." Summer used similar language when she talked about her current sexual relationship, in which they "never, never had sex without a condom," because she viewed condom usage as "a devout practice." In fact, she predicted that her devotion to condom usage would continue for the rest of her life:

> I will never again have sex without a condom unless maybe the man that I marry, wants to have children. And, then only if he understands that [him contracting HPV] is a possibility, or if it were someone who already had HPV . . . I don't know that I'd [have sex without condoms] even then just because the risk [of re-infection] is just too high.

Her words pointed out a difficult reality: Even when both partners shared the same type of STD, re-infection with a new viral strain could occur in the absence of condoms.

For this reason, even women who knew, or had good reason to believe, that their partners were also infected increased their consistency of condom usage. Natasha explained her rationale for practicing safer sex:

> We did use condoms, but then we started not to . . . I had the idea in my head that because he probably was carrying [HPV], and he probably won't show the symptoms, that it was okay. Then I started to think about there being like [many] types of the virus, and so I told him last night, "We need to start using condoms 'cause I don't want to give you anything you don't have, and I don't want you to give me anything I don't have either."

This mindset generally continued until both the women and their infected partners had gone for long periods of time without a new outbreak and committed themselves to monogamous relationships.

When women felt that their partners had been thoroughly tested, and they themselves had been thoroughly treated, concerns like the one expressed above lessened. For example, Pam had a severe case of cervical HPV that progressed to cervical cancer. Her treatments eventually led to her having a hysterectomy at age 38. As her cervix was completely removed, she and her husband did not worry about transmission, but faced different issues. With a shortened vaginal canal and no uterus, Pam noted, "Sex is messier now because there's no place for the semen to go. The first time after [sex], it was sad to see the spills and remember what I'd lost." However, she put a positive spin on her treatment outcome: "[Sex] is also a lot more fun—no condoms or worry about disease or pregnancy."

Guilt

Many of the above women talked about the positive aspects of their new relationships. Summer, the "devout" user of condoms, felt that she "had the most incredible meaningful loving and sexual relationship." However, these new sexual health concerns and practices also produced difficult emotions, such as guilt. This finding parallels Weitz's (1991) research on people living with HIV: "The risk of infecting others forces persons with HIV disease to make adjustments in many of their everyday social interactions and can create further emotional distance and stress in relationships" (102).

Maintaining romantic relationships during times of new outbreaks and treatments often left the women feeling guilty for not being able to feel sexually desirable and be sexually interested in their partners. When Haley recovered from cryosurgery, the "recovery stuff, that month-long discharge that you have to deal with," made her not feel like having sex. While she remembered her partner "being really supportive," and not "pressuring me for anything," she felt bad that her infection had negatively affected their sex life. Likewise, Rhonda's recurrent herpes outbreaks caused her to abstain from sexual relations with her boyfriend. She contended that while, "he was really understanding," her boyfriend also made it clear that "the most difficult part for him was not being able to [have sex]." In spite of feeling guilty, Rhonda has made it a policy to abstain from sex during outbreaks because "it's more dangerous for him, and it's not a comfortable experience for me."

Another aspect of guilt came from the women viewing the negative impacts of their STDs on their current partners and feeling remorse for the sexual behavior that they believe led to their initial infections. Francine explained her emotions:

I felt guilt in bringing this [STD] into the relationship because he had not been anywhere near as sexually active as I had. So, I started feeling remorse for having been so sexually active during the period of time between marriages. He'd been married ten years to somebody else. So, I think I always felt a little more guilty because I might have exposed him to something through my actions.

Rhonda also viewed her herpes as "baggage" she had brought "from another relationship, and it shouldn't have to affect him." Her guilt manifested as feeling "bad sometimes because [herpes] is just kind of thrust upon [my boyfriend]." Similarly, Pam "felt upset, shamed, and guilty" over her "earlier promiscuity." In this manner, the women blamed their own past behaviors for having complicated their current relationships.

Pregnancy

For the women who progressed beyond dating relationships to committed romantic partnerships, issues of pregnancy often became a concern. As discussed in the previous chapter, many of the women who had contracted their STD prior to having children expressed fears of how their infections would affect their fertility and births of future babies. Two of the women in the study had conceived and birthed children while living with both HPV and herpes.

Gloria discussed her experience of being pregnant and delivering her second and third children, after having been diagnosed with herpes, and diagnosed and treated for genital warts:

> I was really concerned because when I had [my second child], no one had ever said to me, "Your baby can catch [warts and herpes] from you if you have an outbreak when you're having the baby." So, when I was having her, I didn't have an outbreak luckily. And, with the third baby, the doctors told me [about the possibilities of transmission and complications], and I was panicked thinking, "What am I gonna' do if I have an outbreak with this baby?"

With her new knowledge, Gloria resolved herself to having a caesarean section, even though she "didn't want to have one . . . if I had an outbreak."[3] She also incorporated education she had gained while receiving treatments and "got very careful about getting rest, not getting too stressed during the ninth months." In the end, she kept her immune system strong and did not have an outbreak during her third pregnancy.

As a professional health educator, Francine used her connections to find a female doctor, who was "really strong in her ob-gyn skills and very alternative" in her approaches to sexual health. Her practitioner took a holistic and long-term approach to Francine's pregnancy: "I actually started going to her before I even got pregnant because we were really planning ahead." With her practitioner's guidance, Francine "did all these really healthy things—made sure my immune system was really strong," both before and during the pregnancy. Francine also appreciated her practitioner's supportive attitude towards Francine's preference for a vaginal birth. Francine remembered her practitioner saying, "Look, we can do this. You can do a vaginal birth. What we'll do is check up until the day you have your baby that there's no herpes present."

With her practitioner's support and encouragement, Francine maintained lifestyle changes, such as giving up coffee, to help stave off herpes outbreaks: "I was just determined that my immune system would be strong. I was so motivated to have a healthy baby, and I really wanted to have a vaginal birth." She ultimately delivered her baby having had no herpes or genital warts outbreaks for the duration of the pregnancy. After giving birth, she recalled thinking "that I'd have outbreaks after the delivery just because I was so exhausted! I thought for sure I'd get outbreaks, and I didn't."

Experiencing Reintegrated Sexual Selves

Those women, who reached a point of sexual-self transformation where they had integrated STD experiences into their intra- and interpersonal lives, reaped the benefits of hard work. Living with a chronic STD had set them off on individualized journeys, all of which seemed to all culminate in a common end: Reintegrated sexual selves. When appropriate, I had included the following questions during the conclusions of interviews:

1. How do you now feel about yourself as a sexual being?
2. Could you share a story that illustrates how you feel about how you have changed?

Personality Traits

The women often told stories of how they felt their personalities had changed. First, some of the women expressed that they had become bolder as a result of their STD experiences. For example, Ingrid shared a story that epitomized her brave new approach to gendered norms of sexual morality. She had attended a sorority dinner where the discussion focused on how a fraternity guy had "lost his virginity" to a "slut:"

This girl said, "Yeah, I heard he had sex with a girl at a party that he didn't know." And she started laughing, and the girl sitting across from me said, "Yeah, she must be some kind of a slut." And I said, "Well, what's your friend Matt?"[4] And she just looked at me, and she goes, "Well, Matt's a really nice guy." And I was like, "Hey, he stuck his penis in her, and he didn't know her. What kind of person is your friend Matt?" And she was, "Well, I guess if you want to put it like that. But this girl must have been a slut."

Ingrid's experiences with contracting an STD had made her question the morality of her own character, and in the end she was determined to take a bold and unpopular stand against the "stereotype that girls are sluts."

Keeping with this theme of courage, several women shared stories about feeling more confident because of illness interactions. In one case, Louise felt that she had become more self-confident about interacting with sexual health practitioners and handling any future health problems that might arise. She envisioned her former self as a "whining person every time I went to the doctor with issues related to my gynecological makeup." For her, "getting over sexual abuse," and managing her cervical HPV infection, had left her "feeling confident about myself, like truly confident." She viewed herself as having overcome "such a huge hurdle" that she felt stronger and more secure. Louise shared her new philosophy: "I think after [surviving sexual abuse and HPV], you just realize that you do have a choice. You choose to confront your problems or you choose to not deal with them. And, everyone has that ability to deal with the problems, if you can figure out how to do it." Having had the tenacity to endure difficult practitioner relationships and several treatments for cervical HPV, Louise had found reason to believe in her ability to successfully handle health problems.

A third change was expressed by many of the women who felt that they had grown to place a higher value on personal integrity in light of their STD interactions. Sierra shared her vision of her sexual future that pointed to another gain: Being able to communicate honestly with sexual partners and put her own health needs first. She commented, "I think in some ways [having HPV] is positive in the sense that it's gonna' force me to be completely honest with somebody up front, and to open up the lines of communication, and take care of myself from the beginning." Her risk awareness had increased to the point that she now viewed all partners as potential health threats "because they very well might have something else." Sierra believed that her new self would not compromise honesty or her health.

Attitudes about Sexual Intimacy

In addition to sharing stories of possessing inner strength, the women also shared new visions of physical intimacy that derived from how they had come to feel about themselves as sexual beings.

For example, Heidi, 31 years old and single at the time of the interview, connected her new comfort with sex to having become comfortable disclosing her STD-status to prospective partners. She summarized, "I became much more comfortable with myself sexually." This comfort came from having altered her priorities within sexual relationships:

> I think it's really become important to me to not jump into sex. In all of my relationships, even the ones where I never had intercourse, I always became physically involved fairly quickly 'cause that's very important to me. But I've also looked back on all my relationships, none of them have worked out, and I don't know if there's a correlation. . . . I mean you certainly don't want to say, "Okay, no physical contact whatever." But, I think it's important to get to a comfort level with someone before you jump into actual sex.

Heidi discovered that slowing down the physically-intimate aspects of a relationship created situations that were less "emotionally damaging" to her sexual self.

Summer discussed a similar discovery: "I realized that sex does not equate to love." In her new approach to intimacy, "a loving relationship should always come first, trust should always come first." She also gained an appreciation for her new vision of herself as a sexual woman: "I'm a woman, and I think women are incredibly beautiful creatures, and that's what I am, and I love myself, and I love my body, and I don't want to just give that to anyone." She now defined sex as "a very special thing," and had no regrets for the traumatic events that had brought her to this realization: "I don't want to be the person I was before."

Other women focused on how their STD experiences had prompted self-discoveries of their sensual and playful sexual selves. Pam, for instance, asserted, "I feel better than ever about myself. When I was a teenager, I hated myself as a sexual being." Having had her husband support her and encourage her to be sexual, after having been treated with a hysterectomy, proved to Pam that she deserved to love her sexual self. Diana expressed similar emotions and expanded on her story of how she was "beginning to develop some sort of erotic self." Like Sierra, she attributed this process to her sexual health status having prompted her to have a more honest and open relationship with a sexual partner:

> I feel like I'm in a stable relationship; I really trust him. It's probably one of the first times I feel like that I'm with somebody that I can really trust . . . I think he really loves and cares for me. So, I can actually sort of explore [my erotic self] a little bit more, and I've been playing around with it. Like sometimes I'll just walk around with a t-shirt on when he's here, and he gets a big kick out of that . . . I'm taking a course on tantric intimacy and have been reading more erotic literature, and just trying to do things that would kind of allow me a chance to do [explore eroticism] in a safe place.

Diana and Pam had both actively helped to create intimate relationships that provided "safe places" for exploring and expanding their sexual possibilities.

The "Big Picture" of STDs

As the women shared their experiences of new sexual selves, they also detailed how living with chronic STDs had influenced how they viewed the larger question of what it meant to have an STD. In different ways, these women had revised their views about a broad range of issues associated with sexual health.

Advocacy was one way that a few of the women chose to disseminate their new views. For example, Summer informally became outspoken amongst her peers, talking about and promoting sexual health awareness. She explained, "I feel like more of an advocate for safe sex, and being aware of your body. There are just things you can't compromise." In a similar vein, Ashley felt that it was important for her to speak out about her condition: "I would have no problem if someone on the street asked me about HPV 'cause I do have it." She contended that she would use such an opportunity to clear up some myths about HPV and tell this hypothetical stranger the following: "It's not anything bad. I'm not gonna' die. I could still have kids. And, if I can have Paps [sic], then I can watch for cervical cancer. I think it sucks, but it took me a long time to realize I'm not a bad person, even though I have this." Ashley and Summer both hoped that others would be able to learn from their examples.

Being a graduate student, Janine, at age 50, had taken a more academic approach to her vision of advocacy. She had come to view STDs "as diseases of reproductive and sexual health" because she thought it was unconstructive to talk "about sex being the cause." She considered herpes and other STDs as having "social causes," and had come to believe that "if you focus on the immoral aspect of [STDs] and sex, then you totally miss the other issues." She viewed the real issue to be the socio-medical climate in which infected individuals were simply assumed to be "promiscuous" and told to "go take a bunch more tests." Janine hoped that her eventual graduate work might lead to better clinical approaches for patients with STDs.

In contrast, more of the women recast STDs in private ways: They internalized beliefs that these diseases were less powerful and less devastating than they had formerly been led to believe. For instance, Ingrid asserted her new standpoint: "Having an STD is not the end of the world . . . my life is not over because of HPV." She believed that more individuals infected with chronic STDs should believe that "they're gonna' be fine." Likewise, Haley expressed, "I've just really grown to deal with [having HPV], and I feel like I'm over it in a way, you know. And that hey, I have it." Changing their views of the "big picture" of STDs helped these women to integrate their illness experiences as positive life lessons.

Reaching the stage of *reintegration* gave these women the sense that they had grown as a result of their illness experiences. They extracted opportunities for introspection and initiated sexual-self "makeovers" that left them feeling stronger in the world. Frank observed a similar phenomenon in his analysis of his own experiences with serious illness: "Illness takes away parts of your life, but in doing so, it gives you the opportunity to choose the life you will lead, as opposed to living out the one you have simply accumulated over the years" (1991,1). Over their years of living with myths of sexual invincibility, STD anxieties, feelings of immorality, challenges of stigma management, and roller-coaster rides of treatment, the majority of the women took pride in how they were living with incurable STDs and in how these illness experiences had changed them for the better.

8 From Personal Tragedies to Social Change

In previous chapters, I described how the lived experiences of incurable STDs transformed women's sexual selves. From analysis of their illness narratives, the following six stages emerged: (1) sexual invincibility, (2) STD anxiety, (3) the immoral patient stage, (4) the damaged goods stage, (5) sexual healing, and (6) reintegration. Several theoretical themes run throughout the women's sexual self transformation processes: Stigma, self and identity, gender, and relationships. In this concluding chapter, I first provide a brief epilogue to the methods section by analyzing the women's reactions to their participation in this research study. Then, I discuss policy and research recommendations for sexual health education and sexual health care. Finally, I examine how the empirical data provide grounds on which to explore how scholarly work on sex, gender, and stigma add to the literature on the self in chronic illness.

Methodological Epilogue

In Chapter 5, I discussed how some of the women used disclosure as an individual stigma management strategy. For many of the women, their interviews with me became cathartic disclosure interactions. As an interested listener, who had no expectations of them aside from hearing their stories, I was a safe person in whom to confide. Also, having been overt about my own STD status and health education experience, the women viewed me as empathetic and useful.

Several of the women mentioned that I was the first person they had ever talked with who also had a chronic STD. For those women who had HPV, I took on the role of being a living example that this disease was "not the end of the world." Summer expressed, "Actually, you're the first person I've ever talked to who I know has [HPV], and it's kinda' nice. It's kinda' reassuring, you know, that there's another human being out there who has [HPV]." Ashley also felt relieved to sit down and talk about her HPV with another person who had lived through similar experiences. She expressed frustration that her previous disclosures had been with individuals who had never heard of HPV before: "No one knew about [HPV], which is amazing." She had seen me give a presentation with the campus sexual health education group and had taken home a flyer I had passed out: "I connected [my HPV] to your class, and I wanted to talk about it so bad 'cause I had never talked with anyone that had it." Since our interview occurred after she had reached reintegration, she reflected that it had been "really difficult not being able to talk to anyone about it, like I kind of went through this on my own, and it took so damn long for me to be okay with it." With women like Summer and Ashley, I observed emotional releases throughout our interviews, with a notable improvement in their moods at the conclusions.

For other women, the act of being interviewed prompted them to ask questions about the medical aspects of their infections: Treatment options, possible outcomes with regard to recurrence frequency, and suggestions of questions they might want to ask their practitioners. Caprice, for example, finished her interview with the following comments:

> Boy, am I glad I talked to you today. Part of the reason I wanted to do the interview was that I wanted to get some of the input. I wanted to hear about some of this. Not like you've given me a ton of information or whatever, but it's kind of nice to talk with someone about it seriously.

I was fortunate to have a follow-up interaction (albeit unplanned) with Caprice who, at the time of our interview, had taken her doctor's advice to forestall having any treatment of her cervical HPV infection. The premise had been to give her body's immune system time to fight the virus. However, at our later encounter, she confirmed that subsequent Pap smears had come back with abnormal test results and she had drawn on our discussion of possible treatment options when it came to talking with her practitioner about pursuing a treatment plan.

The third consequence of using in-depth interviews as a primary method revolved around issues of advocacy and activism. Several of the women noted that I was an HPV-infected woman, who educated others about STDs, and had dedicated her academic work to getting women's STD stories to the attention of scholars, practitioners, and other women experiencing similar health crises. Rhonda, for example, had never participated in any advocacy or activism around her having herpes, but ended our interview with the following offer: "I'm very grateful that you're doing this. I think it's a very wonderful thing, and if there's any way at all that I can help you, keep my number." The research experience gave the participants an opportunity to contribute to an educational cause that had become extremely important to them, while still maintaining their confidentiality.

Policy and Research Recommendations

My ending interview format gave Rhonda and the other participants assurance that I intended for their narratives to be used to help others. I ended every interview with questions that solicited their advice on two related policy issues: Sexual health education and sexual health care of persons with chronic STDs. In this section, I analyze their answers to these questions and link these data to findings from this study, as well as to the work of other researchers.

Sexual Health Education

"What would you want girls to know or learn from your story?" I asked the women. Sometimes, I more specifically asked, "What advice would you have for young women, who haven't yet been diagnosed with an STD, but are having sex?" The women's answers to these questions expanded on themes that have been noted by sexual health researchers

(Leonardo and Chrisler 1992): "Increasing awareness of STDs," "eliminating the double-bind of traditional gender roles," and "social influence and behavioral change" (10–13).

STD Awareness

First, the women attested to the need of increasing general awareness of STDs for adolescents and teenagers. As experienced by the women (in Chapter Two), the American public became much more aware of the possible dangers of sexual activity as a result of HIV/AIDS prevention campaigns. However, education about herpes and HPV had not significantly increased. Monica, for example, remarked on how she had been undereducated about herpes and HPV, both of which can be transmitted via non-penetrative contact. She summarized the lesson she had learned the hard way:

> You can get more [STDs] by doing less than you think you'd have to do. I really think that it's awful that I had to be the example . . . I didn't know that [STDs could be transmitted via] oral sex because I honestly don't know one of my girlfriends that has ever used a condom giving oral sex . . . which is really scary if you think about it.

Since Monica had contracted HPV, via non-penetrative genital-to-genital contact, she was aware of risks posed by the "nontraditional" ways that these two viral infections can be transmitted. From this reference point, she advised sex educators to inform "teenagers and younger people who aren't engaging in sex not to focus on intercourse itself [as the only way to contract an STD] . . . focus on things that people are really doing." Monica wanted teenagers to know about the sexual health risks of oral sex and manual stimulation, and believed that education focusing solely on intercourse gave teenagers a false sense of security when engaging in other sexual behaviors.

Some of the women had additional recommendations for including information beyond STD transmission as part of sex education experiences. Heidi, for instance, specified that sexual health advice would have made more sense to her high-school self if educators had normalized STD testing and had taken the fear out of finding out positive results. She demonstrated how the message should have been presented:

"Don't be afraid to go and get tested and find out for sure because most [STDs] are manageable, even AIDS." Chris also recommended more education on life after STDs: "Let people know that you can control it to some extent with drugs, and you can still be sexually active, even when you have to make adjustments." Heidi and Chris represented a viewpoint that de-stigmatizing STDs would encourage young people to get tested and start to manage their illnesses, rather than fear testing and remain in denial during their first outbreaks.

Overall, the women's recommendations in this area focused on the importance of providing more comprehensive education about the variety of sexual behaviors that can transmit chronic STDs, testing, and the realities of living with STDs.

Gender Roles

The second area of sexual health education concern centered around advice to girls and young women about deviating from traditional gender roles in order to protect themselves from STDs. Researchers have called this issue a "double-bind" because girls/women "are expected to be responsible for the sexual health of the couple, yet they do not have the power to take the necessary action" (Leonardo and Chrisler 1992,12). Haley, for instance, cautioned high school girls to be assertive and openly communicate about sexual health matters:

> My biggest piece of advice for high school girls who are sexually active is to pay attention to who [sic] you're with and get to know them. Get to know their personalities, and if you can't trust them, don't have sex with them . . . they could easily hide something.

Haley's insistence on trust as a key part of high school sexual relationships tied into other women's sentiments on self-respect. For example, Pam emphasized that girls needed to understand their "own worth" and insist on STD examination and testing of partners. Her advice, "Respect yourself," encourages teen girls to value their health over appeasing their partners' desires for sex without testing. In general, the women encouraged gender-role transformations, similar to those they had experienced during reintegration (Chapter 7).

Research on sex education has identified "a gap between the knowledge of sexual risks, intentions, and actual behavior," and some scholars credit this problem to "issues of power, control, masculinity, femininity and sexual identity" (Thomson 1994, 54). The women in my study illustrated some of these issues in their proposed solutions to gaps in sex education. For example, Louise explained, "I think the largest problem with girls in high school is really their self-confidence." In her estimate, "the big issue facing high-school girls is "that a lot of girls get sexually active way too soon in comparison to their emotional health and stability." Having worked with organizations that focus on girls' issues, Louise stated, "I'm always struck by how completely out of touch high-school girls are with their bodies, and yet they're sexually active, and they don't know what they're doing." She wanted sex educators to help girls to explore the gendered reasons why they were deciding to have sex. In this manner, Louise saw the need for curricula to focus on how sex "involves your emotions . . . [because] it's not just a physical activity." In the women's estimations, merely increasing STD awareness would not help girls who felt trapped by their gender roles to passively go along with partners' unhealthy sexual decisions.

Social Influence

The women recognized that given (1) increased STD awareness and (2) educators' encouragements of girls to deviate from feminine sexual-interactional norms (e.g., passivity and other-directedness), the challenge remained to (3) create a social climate that supported sexually healthy behaviors. In this sense, the norms of young women's peers had to be consistent with STD education and prevention recommendations, in order for behavioral change to take place.

Several of the women supported the idea of working to create youth peer norms of sexual responsibility that would extend to teens taking responsibility, both for learning about sexual health issues and for learning about their own sexual health statuses, via medical exams and testing. Summer proposed one way to accomplish this changing of youth values and norms. She proposed that older peers utilize their positions of being admired to educate younger peers about STDs. For example, Summer disclosed her HPV status to her younger sister and brother and told them: "Just wait to have sex. And, if you do, please promise me you'll always, always use protection. Always protect yourself because no person is worth you living with what I'm living with."

Many of the women mirrored this sentiment that "protection" should be the emphasis of both peer and adult sex educators because a sole push for normalizing abstinence left sexually active teenagers uneducated about how to reduce STD risk. In Natasha's opinion, it would have been more effective for her peers to have learned to talk about using condoms and abstaining from riskier behaviors as if it were just another health precaution: "It's just like you're not sharing food with someone who's sick." Kelly asserted that sex educators who emphasized abstinence were not reaching teens with the most realistic and effective message. Rather, she stated, "I would just say it's okay to be sexually active, but if you're gonna' be sexually active, protect yourself." By proposing peer-supported, realistic changes to values and norms, the women's logic was in keeping with the *social influence model* (see Fisher 1988).

Some of the women stressed the importance of destroying the core youth value of sexual invincibility and dismantling stereotypes about persons most likely to contract an STD. For example, Sierra thought young people would have to internalize the following belief in order to make better sexual health decisions: "It doesn't matter who you are or where you came from, who you grew up with, or what kind of environment you grew up in. Anyone can get [HPV], herpes, HIV, or gonorrhea, and you need to be safe." She believed that this message took on more persuasive powers when it came from young people with whom the students could identify. A recent public health study echoes her contention that too many Americans believe that STDs only infect a certain type of person and that this myth impacts our delivery of sexual health services: "STDs are not reserved for a small subset of our society. STDs are equal opportunity infections . . . Routine screening and counseling for these diseases should be the standard of care for all patients in all healthcare settings" (Cline 2006, 357).

The sexual health education policy guidelines, derived from my research, support curricula that begin in elementary school to shape peer norms, so that the peer group will engage in normative processes, such as imposing sanctions on deviant individuals that support STD preventive behaviors and decrease risk. For sexual health education to achieve this larger goal, (1) risk-avoidance behaviors (such as getting tested and using condoms) must be consistent with peer group values, and (2) sexual health peer educators should be trained in order for social influence to appear to come from members of the peer group, and (3) gender norms must change such that girls and boys feel empowered and accountable for making sexually healthy decisions.

Sexual Health Care

In addition to asking the participants how their STD experiences had shaped their opinions of sexual health education, I also asked for what they would like to see changed about sexual health care services, and what they hoped medical practitioners might learn from their lived experiences. These questions generated advice and opinions in the areas of practitioner stance on patient education, practitioner awareness of psychosocial implications of STD diagnoses, and practitioner interaction style.

Patient Education

The women unanimously supported increased patient education as part of diagnostic and treatment sexual health encounters. All wanted sexual health education to be offered explicitly, to be thorough and comprehensive, and to be presented in a considerate manner.

Several explicitly argued that sexual health practitioners had a "responsibility" to educate their patients. Pam, who believed that her "poverty led to my [HPV] getting worse than it had to be," expressed how she would like to remove socioeconomic status as a factor in the quality of sexual health care and education: "I'd tell doctors that poor women deserve treatment, too. Poor women can understand what you tell them, and all women have a right to be well informed."

Lily addressed a different population of women, those who had come of age before schools provided sex education. She believed that this population had been underserved by the school systems and needed more education incorporated into gynecological exams, STD testing, and treatment.

The main point where women will get this information would be at their checkups, their Pap smear at their gynecologist. And I think [practitioners] have a responsibility for educating women. That's something I haven't seen very much of myself. I think they assume at my age that I know stuff. They should understand there's a whole generation of us out there that didn't get this information. We didn't have sexual health educators . . . we just got told how not to get pregnant.

As illustrated in Chapter 2, sexual health education has varied significantly over time, and practitioners may have been operating under false assumptions that all of their patients had received basic STD education during their school years.

Some of the women shared their views of ideal patient education by practitioners. For instance, Deborah focused on the diagnostic exam: "The ideal is education right up front, and, [as a practitioner], you should not be embarrassed to talk about it, or too cursory in your dealings." She emphasized that education was more important for patients diagnosed with viral STDs, like herpes and HPV: "If someone's trying to treat a chronic problem, they should give you the information about how to deal with that."

Other women expounded on why practitioners should focus on education during diagnostic encounters. Haley, for example, wished her practitioner had explained "every detail, like three times" during her diagnostic encounter. Feeling undereducated about HPV, she explained her course of action:

> Left on my own with questions, I called an STD hotline for the technicalities, like how can I spread this to somebody else . . . I'd go back and read the two different kinds of pamphlets on [HPV] that she gave me, and they didn't say exactly when can you and when can't you [transmit the disease] . . . I feel now like I was misinformed: Not informed enough when I was diagnosed.

However, there was a fairly strong consensus among the women that written materials should be a component of patient education. Ashley said, "Basically give [patients] all the information possible." She "didn't even have a little pamphlet or anything" when she left her diagnostic exam. The absence of any written materials resulted in her being "left to sit and think about the warts that were growing on my body."

The above stories pointed to a basic flaw in many practitioners' approaches to patient education: A lack of assessing patients' sexual health knowledge levels before presenting information. Rhonda, for example, presented an alternative mindset that could help with this problem:

> Understand that the person who you're [presenting a diagnosis] to has no idea what you're saying. They don't know what you're talking about and what it means. We go to doctors because they're supposed to be the experts on this, and they should be able to tell you what's going on and what's gonna' happen.

Rhonda contended that practitioners should view themselves as being "responsible for preparing" patients for the treatment plans and lifestyle changes that chronic STDs demand of those infected.

Key to this preparation, women argued, practitioners needed to provide detailed information about both medical and interpersonal issues connected with having chronic STDs. Several of the women thought that this need would best be served by an additional, post-diagnostic appointment. Sandy, for example, described setting up "strictly an information session" about the particular STD. In this setting, she envisioned that the practitioner would talk about "everything." This session should include information about transmission: "How to protect yourself and how to protect other people from getting it." In addition, Sandy hoped this type of session would allow patients to gain better understandings of the extent of their infection: She wanted to know "specifically what my symptoms are right now, like do I have warts on the inside, 'cause I know I don't have them on the outside, or right now do I have nothing?" In general she made an argument that patients "need to know specifics, details," if they were to feel like their conditions were manageable.

Heidi suggested a similar post-diagnostic scenario, in which patients could share their concerns and ask questions. She, too, thought that medical issues of transmission would need to be clarified, " 'cause I worried, 'Can this be transmitted through oral sex?' " In addition, she foresaw the need for patients to get advice on interpersonal issues, such as disclosure: "What exactly should I tell my partner about this?

How can I reassure him that it's not a big deal?" Researchers have agreed that STDs, as public health epidemics, would best be decreased when patients were well educated and adjusted their sexual behavior to reduce the risks of transmission (Keller et al. 1995; Leonardo and Chrisler 1992). How can this goal be accomplished? Ideally, the focus and style of medical training would change to incorporate more holistic goals of patient care, including educating patients about the medical and social aspects of their illnesses. Research has shown that "humanistic training" of student physicians has been partly responsible for a shift away from views of authority in physician-patient relationships that support the traditional "medical model" of interaction (Lavin et al. 1987). However, professional and economic constraints have made it likely for the medical model of practitioner interaction style to remain dominant. Thus, professional health educators should be added to the medical team. They would be able to provide not only education about symptoms and treatment options, but also emotional/psychological support that would complement the technical expertise provided during practitioner interactions.

Psychosocial Implications of Diagnoses

Data presented in Chapter 5 revealed psychosocial implications for women being diagnosed with chronic STDs. From an applied standpoint, this study adds the sociological dynamics of stigma to the factors practitioners should consider when presenting STD diagnoses. While the previous section detailed Haley's request for better patient education at diagnostic encounters, she admitted that more education at that point in time might not have done her the most good: "I might have been so overwhelmed by [the diagnosis] that I kind of missed things that she was telling me." Her assessment reflects the way that the emotional fallout of the psychosocial aspects of STDs must be considered in sexual health care recommendations.

These extra-medical components of STDs became important to the women's assessments of how health care delivery could be improved. As illustrated by Natasha's recollection of her emotional state, when receiving her genital warts diagnosis: "I was pretty shaken up—I couldn't really ask questions at that point." She concluded her interview with the following advice for practitioners:

Make sure the first time that you tell 'em that it's more like a counseling visit than just like stating the facts because the diagnosis of STD can be very crucial to people. People think only AIDS can be devastating because it can kill you, but it's important to counsel all people because all STDs are tough, especially ones that are long term, not curable.

Caprice expanded on this issue by suggesting that practitioners offer written materials (e.g., pamphlets) at the diagnostic encounter because she, too, "didn't want to hear" what her practitioner had to say at that moment in time. She remembered, "I almost stopped to ask [for a pamphlet on HPV], and I felt kind of silly . . . I was looking at the racks on the wall, saw something about HPV, and I should have just asked. But, because it wasn't offered to me, I didn't make that extra step." She would have appreciated her practitioner or a clinic staff person giving her printed materials to take home, so that she "could refer to it later."

Some of the women had had positive experiences with practitioners, who understood the multiple layers of meaning within a chronic STD diagnosis. Sierra appreciated how her practitioner had allowed her the space to process the non-medical aspects of her diagnosis and then helped to make her feel better:

One thing that was good was that my health practitioner left the room after she told me [my diagnosis and went] to get the treatment kit. But, I think she kind of left [for a] longer [period of time] than she needed to, just to give me a minute to regroup and feel what I was feeling. And I think that was really good. I mean I think she gave me a moment to kind of absorb it, and then she came back in, and I was crying . . . I think she tried to tell me a story about someone else who had it and reassured me that I'm not the only one with it, which was nice to hear.

Overall, Sierra felt that "being gentle and respecting that people are gonna' have intensive reactions is really important."

Researchers have found support for the idea that practitioners need to understand STDs as multi-faceted diseases in order to provide optimal care. One study found that patients had a high likelihood of becoming upset upon learning that they have an STD and consequently felt shame and embarrassment (Keller et al. 1992). A follow-up study determined that this type of reaction left patients with impaired capabilities for absorbing important medical information passed on by practitioners during a diagnostic interaction (Keller et al.1995, 359):

> These emotional responses can block an individual's ability to take in further information about the disease and its treatment. If this appears to be the case, another appointment strictly for purposes of counseling and education, is indicated. The content of any counseling and education intervention depends partly on the needs expressed by the client. Thus, it is very important to assess the meaning the individual assigns to the infection.

The data provided in Chapter 4 illustrate the above point by showing how patients can be preoccupied and devastated by the impact of multiple stigma during diagnostic encounters. Protocol for patient care should be informed by research on the emotional impact of diagnoses and the ways in which patients assess and assign meanings to their illnesses.

Practitioner Interaction Style
The data also point to a correlation between practitioners' understandings of STDs and social and psychological phenomena and their interaction styles: Greater levels of understanding may produce kinder interaction styles, and vice versa. Rhonda illustrated this connection with her advice to practitioners: "Treat [a patient] like [she] was your own child: Don't just say, 'Okay, this is what you have. It's been really nice seeing you. Get out.' Be sensitive and understand that it's probably really a traumatizing thing to find out." Sensitivity during diagnostic and treatment interactions was one of the women's most frequent recommendations.

Those women, who had enjoyed their practitioner interactions, explained the qualities that they had perceived as beneficial and that they believed would help other women in similar situations. For example, Elle contended that there was nothing she had wished that her practitioner had done differently in diagnosing and treating her herpes infection. She stated, "The person I got the diagnosis from was very normalizing and very optimistic," and she believed other women would benefit from this type of practitioner demeanor. Similarly, Summer described a practitioner who treated her with respect and made her feel comfortable getting her questions answered:

> I called this woman . . . I'll never forget her, God rest her soul. She talked to me and made me feel so much better . . . You know, she had me laughing and just feeling so much better about myself. And so she mailed me all of this stuff: A big package of folders.

Putting patients at ease, giving them hope for the future, and welcoming any questions were the top qualities of favored practitioners. Ashley summarized what almost of the women expressed wanting from their practitioner interactions: "Just let [patients] know that it's not the end of the world, like this [STD] is okay. It can be taken care of."

However, many of the women were dissatisfied with their practitioners' bedside manners, and they recommended changes in this area when asked how practitioners might improve patient care. For example, Cleo, whose practitioners gave her an HPV diagnosis without explaining that it was sexually transmitted, would have appreciated if a staff person had initiated interactions to make sure that she understood it was an STD. She imagined that a practitioner with a warmer interaction style would have helped her to express her feelings and ask questions:

> It would have been nice if there had been somebody I'd been comfortable enough to ask, "Well, it is a sexually transmitted disease, right?" . . . There were a lot of feelings. Probably at the time, I would have had a lot of things to talk about, the fact that it was my first partner, about how it made me feel so ashamed, and about feeling guilty about having sex with other partners.

Sierra, similarly criticized the "health care industry" for having a "rush, rush, rush, gotta get in, get out" mentality. She expressed a desire for system-wide changes to reduce the number of patients who "aren't being taken care of in a holistic sense, in that they're not being talked to about all the things that could be affecting what is going on with them."

Other women made a point of how their practitioners' physical interactions had made them uncomfortable. Kelly, for instance, had a female doctor who pulled up her examination gown to take her heart rate, and this action caught Kelly completely off-guard. "I would just let her know I like to be told exactly what you're doing before you're going to do it to me, and that way I'll know rather than be surprised." In general, she believed that practitioners should "be aware of what [patients] want and what it would take to make [patients] feel comfortable." Similar complaints and recommendations were voiced by many of the women.

Women's recommendations for increased respect also extended to issues of morality. This study points to the possibility of practitioner interaction style influencing patient interactions, such that stigma and shame became a part of medical interactions. If public health is the goal, then practitioners must safeguard the moral identities of patients. The women appreciated practitioners who interacted with them as if they were blind to stereotypes of women with STDs. In contrast, women who had interacted with judgmental practitioners, made pointed critiques and requests for revised interaction styles. Natasha presented her assessment:

> [Practitioners] should provide [encouragement for] being protected during sex, but not necessarily make people feel wrong for sleeping with some certain number [of partners] or [feel] that sex is bad. [Practitioners] may not mean to [inspire] that feeling, but often it comes out that way.

Her objection reflected a common objection against practitioners, who interacted with patients in ways that displayed moral contempt or assumptions of moral impropriety on the parts of the patients. Medical researchers on STDs have argued, "Once the diagnosis is understood, provision of sensitive, nonjudgmental, supportive care is critical" (Keller et al. 1995, 359).

Survey research has supported the finding that "patients rely heavily on the physician's mode of communicating when evaluating the care delivered by the physician" (Buller and Buller 1987). Practitioner interaction style is an important determinant of patient satisfaction with both practitioner and medical treatment (Daly and Hulka 1975; Korsch et al. 1968; Spiro and Heidrich 1983). From a public health perspective, this issue gained importance in light of findings that compliance appeared to be largely a result of patient satisfaction (Korsch et al. 1968; Korsch and Negrete 1972, Woolley et al. 1978).

In the case of the moralistic practitioners, there are public health risks, in the form of patient compliance and emotional well-being, of social and professional acceptance of this interaction style. Not only my study, but also research on HIV counseling and treatment, have suggested that protecting the moral status of the patient is key in obtaining compliance (Plumridge and Chetwynd 1998). Through adjustments to practitioner-patient interaction styles, society may be able to produce patients who are more likely to follow medical treatment plans and modify risky behaviors because they not only have better understandings of medical pathways toward healing, but they also believe that they deserve to get well.

Additionally, we need to push for increased funding of sexual health education programs and health care services. "STD and HIV/AIDS programs at the state and local levels remain highly controversial, lack strong public approval, are significantly underfunded, and are frequently fractured at service delivery points" (Cline 2006, 357). STD epidemics will continue to spread throughout our communities until we succeed in de-stigmatizing, not only the diseases, but more importantly, the infected individuals. We can only achieve this by increasing the public's awareness about the accurate risks of acquiring STDs, and by increasing our openness to discussing the full range of consequences—social, psychological, economic—that impact the infected, their sexual partners, and their children. While a cure for HSV and HPV may not be yet in our grasp, there is nothing to stop us from changing social norms and values in ways that will improve the everyday experiences of the unnamed millions, whose lives are often more damaged by STD-related stigma—the shame, guilt, fear, depression, and anxiety—than by the viruses themselves.

STD Stigma in Action—The Truth behind the "Cervical Cancer" Vaccine

Has the renaming and reframing of the HPV vaccine into the cervical cancer vaccine eliminated the public's concerns about making this vaccine available (and potentially funded by federal programs and mandated by states) to adolescent and teen girls? Let's take the case of New Hampshire. In January 2007, this state became the first to add GARDASIL to its childhood vaccination program: It is offered to girls, between the ages of 11 and 18 years old, as part of a state program that offers many immunizations to children for free. This program is paid for by insurance companies and the federal government. However, there is already a shortage in this state: Waitlists are growing.

According to an article from New Hampshire, in the *Concord Monitor* (Sanger-Katz 1/7/07): "Doctors say few parents have been uncomfortable with the idea of giving such young children a vaccine for a sexually transmitted disease." This article went on to quote pediatrician Dr. Suzanne Boulter: "I've been shocked that I've had parents just asking me over and over again [to vaccinate their daughters]." She expressed disappointment over the vaccine shortage, citing that the forty-three doctors at her office will receive only fifteen doses per month. Dr. Boulter gave her explanation for the popularity of this new vaccine: "I think parents can separate their daughters being sexually active from cancer prevention." She is partially correct. Parents might be able to separate HPV vaccination from sexual activity because it has been sold to them as a *cancer* vaccine.

While it may seem to make sense to have achieved a greater public good by having the American public believe that the first HPV vaccine is a cervical cancer vaccine, what are the ramifications of this social construction, with regard to public health? What are the dangers of the American public believing that (1) HPV causes all cervical cancer and (2) disassociating HPV from the category of infectious diseases known to be sexually transmitted?

Limitations of HPV Vaccination

HPV is an epidemic that continues to baffle the medical community. There is no cure for HPV, no agreement on prevention strategies for sexually-active individuals, and no approved tests for HPV infection in male or female patients, except for the cervical cancer screening that is part of a Pap smear (Friedman and Shepeard 2007). So, what do we know about GARDASIL? It is designed to be given in three doses over a six-month time period. Studies have shown it to be safe and effective: "at least five years of safety data that include no hints of long-term risks or waning effectiveness. But if the vaccine should begin to lose potency over time, that could easily be remedied by a booster shot" (Brody 2007). While approved for women up to 26 years-old, it is considered best, if administered to girls between the ages of 9 to 13, with the hope of reaching them before sexual activity potentially exposes them to HPV.[1] Since the vaccine against HPV is targeted to preadolescent children, parental acceptance of this vaccine is critical for its success. However, "the HPV vaccine is no magic bullet: It has the potential to substantially reduce the prevalence of cervical cancer, but not to eradicate it" (Parry 2007, 89).

How will the cost of this vaccine impact its effectiveness? Can this medical intervention ever be truly accessible to the variety of girls and women who could benefit from it? The three-dose vaccination schedule of GARDASIL has been estimated to cost approximately $120 per dose in the U.S.: "this high cost might mean that some socioeconomic groups in the United States will remain unvaccinated" (Honey 2006, 3087). Even with GARDASIL now covered by the Vaccines for Children Program (that provides free immunizations to children with Medicaid coverage, American Indian and Alaska Native children), some U.S. girls and young women will not qualify for this program and have neither health insurance, nor the funds to pay for the vaccine themselves. In addition, we must figure out how to address the challenge of vaccinating young immigrants, especially those who are undocumented and may be ineligible for public health programs. Over half of the deaths from cervical cancer in the U.S. have occurred in foreign-born women (Seeff and McKenna 2003). Many are optimistic that the benefits will ultimately outweigh the financial costs and difficulties that face those creating HPV vaccine policies and practices, as the annual expenses of cervical cancer in the U.S. have been estimated to range from $181.5 million to $363 million.[2]

Some have raised a concern about a HPV vaccine triggering "behavioral disinhibition" among vaccinated adolescents. The fear is that those who are vaccinated will incorrectly believe that they face no health dangers from sex and, therefore, they will become sexually active earlier than they would have otherwise and increase unsafe sexual activities (increase their number of partners, increase the variety of sexual behaviors, etc.). This concern only makes sense if one believes that adolescents' awareness of HPV, and fear of contracting HPV, are their primary motivations for abstinence and/or safer sex. Research studies have found the contrary to be true: That the American public (male and female adolescent and adult populations) has an extremely low awareness of HPV as a sexually transmitted disease (Raine et al. 2005; Smoak et al. 2006). According to the Family Research Council's (FRC) online statements, they accept Merck's claim that studies have shown that "sexual disinhibition" is not an outcome of this vaccine; though, they urge Merck to reexamine this issue after the vaccine has been more widely distributed (FRC 2007a).

The CDC's 2003 focus group study explored this issue by raising questions about "whether perceptions of immunity would reduce condom use by vaccinated individuals, thereby increasing their risk for other STDs. Strong concerns were voiced by [the participants who were] parents about giving children a false sense of security and implicitly condoning unsafe or promiscuous youth sexual behaviors" (Friedman and Shepeard 2007, 8). These are the same reasons that many state and local boards of education have opted for abstinence-until-marriage sex education policies (Cline 2006).

The FRC still strongly opposes states making this a mandatory vaccine for school attendance (2007a). State legislation mandating the HPV vaccine will allow parents to opt out for "medical, moral, or philosophical reasons. This opt-out clause might be used more often than for other mandatory vaccines, as some critics feel that because HPV is a sexually transmitted disease, providing the vaccination to girls before they become sexually active endorses underage sex and promiscuity" (Honey 2006:3087). However, the FRC aims to convince all states to make it an "opt-in" vaccine, which would entail that parents of adolescent girls and young women (18 to 26 years old) would have to request the vaccine from their medical practitioners, rather than it being offered as one of the already standardized vaccines (FRC 2007b).

A recent article in the health section of *The New York Times* reframes this issue and challenges the FRC's stance: "In response to suggestions of mandatory HPV vaccination for all girls entering high school, opponents have objected to 'forcing' therapy on healthy girls under the presumption that future behavior might result in disease. This is exactly the principle on which every form of immunization is based" (Brody, accessed online May 21, 2007). It is interesting to note that, historically, there was not a similar outcry over the May 2001 FDA licensing of *Twinrix*, a vaccine that offers combined protection against both hepatitis A and hepatitis B, even though both of these viruses are most commonly transmitted via sexual behaviors and injection drug use (Cline 2006). So, perhaps the CDC and Merck had it right all along: As long as Americans are uneducated about the sexually-transmitted nature of a virus, they will not likely protest a vaccine for that virus being state-funded with an "opt-out" policy for adolescents.

The FRC also wants a clear message about the limitations of the vaccine (and the benefits of abstinence) to accompany all marketing and educational materials about GARDASIL. The CDC's own study concurs: "Accurate and reliable health information is needed to inform the public, particularly women and parents of vaccine-eligible girls, about HPV-associated risk, interpreting cervical cancer screening results, and managing and treating [pathologies related to prior HPV infection]" (Friedman and Shepeard 2007, 3).

There are compelling reasons for states to mandate an HPV vaccine, along with other standard pre-teen vaccinations. Adding a HPV vaccine to state's childhood vaccination programs is partly an effort of STD destigmatization. Experts on biological therapies argue that, "Giving the HPV vaccine at the same time as the other preteen vaccinations . . . would place the vaccine in the scope of preventative medicine and possibly remove any social stigma. Another advantage to vaccinating adolescents is that children 10–15 years old have a stronger immune response than those who are 16–23 years old" (Dinh and Benoit 2007, 482).

In addition, abstinence-until-marriage sex education has become the norm in the U.S. over the past two decades. Even though academic researchers across disciplines concur that ". . . the abstinence message is rarely effective. Half of all girls become sexually active before graduating from high school" (Brody 2007). Due to the prophylactic nature of this vaccine, it must be given prior to "exposure" (i.e., sexual activity). As the behaviors of early initiation of sexual activity and multiple sex partners have become normalized in recent decades, adolescents are viewed as the best candidates for a vaccine that must be given before a young person's "debut" of sexual activity.

In addition, even the FRC agrees with health and sexuality researchers that vaccinating adolescent girls is necessary because, even if they are abstinent, they may not be able to avoid nonconsensual sex (rape, incest, etc.). Given the lack of comprehensive sex education, the absence of well-funded public health campaigns about STDs in the U.S., and the dominant *myth of sexual invincibility*, it makes sense to target any STD vaccine at this age group: "Adolescents are at increased risk because of their risk-taking behaviors and lack of awareness about HIV/STDs" (Cline 2006, 355).

Is this a Case of Reverse Sexism?

Anybody who knows anything about reproductive anatomy can figure out that boys and men do not have cervixes; therefore they are not at risk for cervical cancer, so why would they need a "cervical cancer" vaccine? There will be no way to promote GARDASIL and other HPV vaccines to adolescent boys and men without a new campaign to clarify that this is an HPV vaccine and that HPV is a sexually transmitted disease. To date, the CDC claims that they do not yet know if the vaccine is effective in boys or men. On their website, they have issued the following statement: "It is possible that vaccinating males will have health benefits for them by preventing genital warts and rare cancers, such as penile and anal cancer. It is also possible that vaccinating boys/men will have indirect health benefits for girls/women" (CDC 2006).

The current gender-biased policy, and lack of completed research of the vaccine on boys and men, seems to support the gendered double-standard of sexual morality. The policies appear to continue to treat girls and women as the "vectors and vessels" of HPV (Davidson 1994; Luker 1998; Mahood 1990). Some have made the seemingly practical argument that if all the girls and women are vaccinated, the disease will also cease to exist among boys and men. That logic relies on the heterosexist assumption that all boys and men will choose to have female partners. It also discounts the desires of parents of boys, boys, and young men themselves, to prevent themselves from becoming infected with strains of a virus that have been proven to have serious health risks. In boys and men, the same types of HPV that have been linked to cervical cancer can cause cancer of the penis, urethra, anus, and a subset of oral, head and neck cancers. Research has shown that HPV vaccination of male adolescents may be beneficial because genital warts, penile cancer, and anal cancer are also HPV-related diseases (Partridge and Koutsky 2006). In addition, a gender-neutral approach to HPV-vaccination would have a larger impact in a shorter amount of time. A 2007 report from the American Cancer Society[3] notes that vaccination of males may be recommended to prevent, not only anogenital warts in males and the subset of cancers mentioned above, but also the indirect infection of their female and/or male sexual partners and juvenile respiratory papillomatosis in their children.

The American Academy of Family Physicians endorses practitioner-initiated discussions of substance use, obesity/physical activity, and sexual health. The new HPV vaccination could jumpstart these conversations. Unfortunately, as Temte (2007) notes, "The potential benefit of this starting point is reduced, however, because the prevention and anticipatory guidance is targeted only at girls . . . there is need to further evaluate the effectiveness of this vaccine in males, and to thoughtfully develop a routine early adolescence preventive health care visit for both sexes in family medicine settings" (30).

In developing countries, "The most successful vaccination programmes [sic] have been community-wide and avoid any stigma associated with single-sex vaccination, but the cost may restrict HPV vaccination to girls, especially since clinical data on efficacy on boys are still being gathered" (Parry 2007, 89). Experts believe this to be true in the U.S. as well, and efficacy trials of the GARDASIL vaccine on adolescent boys and young men are expected to conclude some time in 2008.

Factors Found to Influence the Acceptance of HPV Vaccination

The CDC, recognizing the potential power of STD-related stigma to affect the American public's acceptance of a HPV vaccine, had the foresight to conduct a 2003 focus group study of 25 to 45 year-old adults in six cities throughout the U.S. The goal of this research was to explore individuals' beliefs, attitudes, and knowledge about HPV and about a hypothetical vaccine, since no real vaccine had been licensed yet by the FDA. So, what made these adults confused and concerned about having their adolescent girls and young women vaccinated? "This STD-associated stigma, in addition to participants' lack of knowledge about HPV, precluded the groups from reaching any consensus on the appropriate age of vaccination or whether to incorporate the vaccine into routine childhood immunizations" (Friedman and Shepeard 2007, 8). STD-related stigma and lack of knowledge about HPV are recurrent themes in recent studies, which have looked at what affects how parents, young women, and medical practitioners perceive the acceptability of a HPV vaccine.

Similar to my study's findings, the CDC researchers found that male and female participants mentioned the following words when asked what they associated with the term *sexually transmitted disease* or *STD*: "promiscuity," "infidelity," "shame," "embarrassment," "guilt," and "divorce" (Friedman and Shepeard 2007:5). These same researchers cautioned about the negative power of STD stigma: "We must disconnect HPV from notions of promiscuity and stigma. This could have important implications for cervical cancer screening practices and vaccine uptake" (Friedman and Shepeard 2007:13). If public campaigns fail to dismantle the STD stereotype of promiscuity, then health officials fear we will not see enough individuals who are married or involved in non-marital committed relationships getting vaccinated: "A lack of perceived susceptibility to HPV emerged as a barrier to vaccine acceptability" (Friedman and Shepeard 2007, 7). Only by promoting more accurate understandings of HPV risks will a vaccine campaign achieve its maximum impact.

A 2006 study (Dempsey et al.) found that providing parents with an information sheet on HPV increased knowledge about the disease; however, this improvement in knowledge had negligible effects on the parents' view of HPV vaccines as acceptable for their children. Rather, this research revealed that parents' life experiences and attitudes proved to be more significant factors in shaping their determination of HPV vaccine acceptability. Attitudes about STDs and sexual morality have also proven to be key in predicting young women's views about receiving a HPV vaccine. Variables associated with young women's acceptability of HPV vaccination include not only "knowledge about the disease," but also "belief that others would approve of the vaccination" (Dinh and Benoit 2007, 482). There still is a strong fear that others will judge a person to be promiscuous if they seek a vaccine to protect them from an STD. All of the research highlights how the case of the HPV vaccine underscores the argument that the de-stigmatization of all sexually transmitted diseases is truly needed to achieve improved public health in the U.S.

The Larger Context of U.S. STD Education and Public Health Campaigns

Research conducted prior to the advent of GARDASIL reveals that medical practitioners, HPV and cervical cancer researchers, and public health advisors have warned that a campaign to promote a HPV vaccine, which focused primarily on the sexually transmitted nature of HPV, would risk stigmatizing the vaccine and jeopardize the success of addressing cervical cancer– viewed to be a more important public health issue. (Braun and Gavey 1999; CDC 2002). Given the current pharmaceutical campaign to promote GARDASIL, it is clear that Merck heeded these cautions and took into account that they would have to contend with different public attitudes depending upon whether they chose to frame HPV primarily as a cause of cervical cancer, as an STD, or as a general public health concern. Their choice has been clear: There is a national public health campaign to promote the "cervical cancer vaccine" and no similar efforts to educate the public about HPV, an STD of epidemic proportions for both sexes.

There is reason to believe that this strategy may backfire in promoting vaccine acceptance. A 2003 focus-group study, commissioned by the CDC's Division of STD Prevention, found that "Audience awareness and knowledge of HPV were low across all groups. This, along with an apparent STD-associated stigma, served as barriers to participants' hypothetical acceptance of a future vaccine." (Friedman and Shepeard 2007:1). A more explicit public health campaign about HPV would not only increase the number of U.S. women and men who know what HPV is, and its link to cervical cancer, it could also clarify that carcinogenic HPV types do not only affect the cervix. In addition to the previously noted consequences for boys and men, these HPV types can also cause vulvar, urethral, and anal cancers in girls and women. The CDC's study supports the American public's desire for a more complete education on this topic. "Participants generally wanted factual, current information about the nature of HPV and its link to cancer; methods of transmission, prevention, and detection; and the treatment of its symptoms and consequences" (Friedman and Shepeard 2007, 10).

But, what about the anxiety created by new knowledge about cervical cancer and HPV for sexually active adults who, by virtue of age or other factors, do not have access to the vaccine? Given my findings, I think that a realistic dose of HPV education could go a long way towards dismantling the *myth of sexual invincibility*. The anxiety could be addressed by a campaign to normalize HPV, perhaps via statistics, and to demystify the health consequences and treatment options. Some have noted that increased awareness of HPV is likely to provoke a desire for HPV testing among women and men, and researchers caution that public demand for HPV DNA testing could "lead to inappropriate use of the test and higher health care costs . . . it also could label and possibly stigmatize healthy individuals as diseased, when they are merely carriers of a virus that is likely to resolve on its own without clinical consequence" (Friedman and Shepeard 2007, 11).

While it makes sense to keep health care costs in check, I am troubled by this presumption that medical practitioners and clinical researchers know best what each of us, with our unique life experiences, might want or even need to know about our sexual health statuses. All measures should be taken to prevent any unwarranted public hysteria over HPV. Educational media campaigns and printed materials should make it clear the majority of new HPV infections do not cause serious medical problems and do become clinically undetectable within one year. But, using STD-related stigma as a reason to discourage HPV DNA testing, or other STD-screenings, does not make for good public health policy.

The Future of GARDASIL and other STD Vaccines

GARDASIL may be the first HPV vaccine licensed by the FDA, but it will certainly not be the last. In March 2007, GlaxoSmithKline formally asked the FDA to approve its Cervarix vaccine, which protects against only the types (16 and 18) associated with precancerous cervical lesions. Others are currently working on vaccines for HSV (herpes simplex virus) and, of course, there is great support for finding a HIV vaccine.

HPV and cervical cancer are global issues. The World Health Organization (WHO) recently issued recommendations on introducing HPV vaccines to other countries. Their guidelines "drive home the need to educate governments, health professionals and the public about both viruses and vaccines, and the importance of collaboration between reproductive health, immunization, child and adolescent health, and cancer control programmes [sic]" (Parry 2007, 89).

The acceptance issues facing any STD vaccine include the acceptance by medical practitioners. Zimet (2006) explained two factors that must be addressed and improved upon in order to enable health care professionals to play a positive role in the success of a HPV vaccination campaign: "Physician comfort with recommending a human papillomavirus vaccine to women and parents of preadolescents; and physician communication skills related to talking with women and parents about the vaccine" (23). As my data and other studies have shown, knowledge about HPV varies significantly among health care providers. Providers most likely to be involved with HPV vaccinations will be pediatricians and primary care providers who, unlike gynecologists, may have limited understanding or familiarity with HPV.

Eng and Butler (1997) suggest that Americans' reluctance to address STDs openly is a result of not only biological, but also social factors. But, Americans are not alone in promoting a stigmatizing silence around the topic of sexual disease. By the end of 2006, forty-nine countries around the world had approved a HPV vaccine (WHO 2007), and that number is expected to increase in the coming year. Fear, embarrassment, anxiety, inadequate knowledge, misperception of risk, religious beliefs—these shape how individuals and governments around the world are addressing topics like the HPV vaccine. STDs, including HIV, are serious global public health problems, and vaccines, while a powerful preventive medical tool, cannot be utilized to their full potential as long as STD-related stigma persist. It is vital that we prioritize funding to collaborate across communities in the U.S., and with leaders around the world, to develop STD de-stigmatization campaigns that are sensitive to issues of social context (sex, gender, race, ethnicity, social class, age, etc.). This might be effective in changing the social norms and values that, not only damage the lives of those infected, but also make it more difficult to halt the spread of sexually transmitted pandemics.

The Gendered Self in Chronic Illness

Gender provides an overarching lens through which to examine theoretical issues of stigma, self, identity, and relationships. Taking a first-hand experiential perspective, this research study fills some gaps in scholarly understandings of the role played by gender in shaping social psychological implications of chronic STD transmission, diagnosis, and treatment. In addition, my findings test and expand theoretical models of stigma, identity crisis, stigma management, and deviant identity formation.

Gender and the Stigma of STDs

This book highlights how the discourses that shape sexual health practices serve to embody and reaffirm social patterns of gender subordination. Sexuality has been "socially organized and critically structured by gender inequality" (Walby 1990, 121). My study points to the fact that sexual health interactions are also shaped by gender norms and inequality. A comparable study of men with chronic STDs would be able to test whether the degree to which patients perceive STD diagnoses as moral and tribal stigma is dependent upon their internalized gender norms of sexual morality. Sarah, a graduate student with HPV, mirrored findings of the African AIDS researchers cited in the introduction: "I don't think STDs are pleasant for men, but they can be a badge of honor in that they represent the ability to have a lot of sexual partners." Even Elle, the one woman who experienced minimal tribal stigma, did not perceive any social benefits as having resulted from her contracting an incurable STD.

Medical views have historically portrayed the female body as "unclean, weak, and ill;" their assertions have served as the basis for representing women "as the source of sexually transmitted diseases, a view which served to validate the sociocultural image of woman as dangerous" (Leonardo and Chrisler 1992, 2). Gilman's (1988) historical discussion of syphilis describes how, "the individual bearing the signs and stigmata of syphilis [became] that of the corrupt female" (254). My data confirm the significance of this sex-based double standard (for sexual morality and sexual health) in understanding how women try to make sense of their own STD diagnoses.

Illness Stigma and Identity Crises

This work explores the confluence of morality and medicine. Diagnosed as "immoral patients," the women experienced Goffman's (1963) three types of stigma: Abomination of the body, blemish of character, and tribal stigma. STD diagnoses stigmatized the women's sexual bodies, moral characters, and social statuses. In turn, the women confronted identity dilemmas of who they were, in terms of being diseased and contagious, perceived as immoral (by self and others), and demoted to an unsavory social caste.

Variations of the three stigma and corresponding identity crises have been described and analyzed by those who have researched individuals living with HIV/AIDS (Sandstrom 1998; Tewksbury and McGaughey 1997; Weitz 1991). However, only one study (Grove et al. 1997) examined a sample of women who were HIV-seropositive and possessed levels of status, or "symbolic capital" (Bourdieu 1986), that were similar to the women I interviewed. Their study of women with wealth, status, and educational attainment found that subjects experienced HIV/AIDS without the blemish of character or tribal stigma. "In the public discourse surrounding HIV/AIDS, the fact that these women can be labeled as innocent victims speaks volumes" (Grove et al. 1997, 319). The researchers attributed the ability of these women to continue to see themselves as "nice girls" to the social construction of AIDS as being linked to social groups so different from their own: Gay men, intravenous drug users, racial minorities, and the lower classes.

In contrast, my research shows that even women with high levels of symbolic capital may see themselves—and believe that others will perceive them—as "bad girls," responsible for their own infections. In contrast to those interviewed by Grove et al. (1997), none of the women I interviewed drew "on the cultural dichotomy between 'us' (nice girls) versus 'them' (outsiders)" (334) to guard themselves against tribal stigma. Aside from Elle, all of the women, regardless of their actual levels of sexual experience, felt that being diagnosed with incurable STDs branded them as "bad girls."

Why would there be this difference between women's illness experiences of HIV/AIDS versus chronic STDs? Researchers found that the HIV-seropositive women with symbolic capital were "neither discredited nor morally contaminated" (Grove et al. 1997, 335). Their finding posits a link between being able to avoid social discrediting and being able to avoid the blemishing of character. Drawing on Goffman's (1963) differentiation between *the discredited* and *the discreditable*, the only setting in which the women I studied were explicitly discredited was in the doctor's office, where their records contained documentations of diagnoses, treatments, and follow-up exams. The women with internal/cervical HPV were able to "pass" for healthy even when naked and engaged in sexual intercourse. The women with external HPV and genital herpes were able to "pass" when asymptomatic. Given the potential to remain discreditable in most relationships, why did they experience blemish of character and tribal stigma?

I credit these differences to the specific socio-historical construction of non-HIV STDs as especially stigmatizing to women, such that gender as a master status interacts with the auxiliary traits of being sexually diseased. The "STD-infected" master health status stigmatizes a woman both morally and socially. My research supports Lock's (2000) idea of medical agents acting in the best interest of the socially dominant (men, in the case of STDs): "It is with special emphasis on ethnicity and gender differences, that the well-being of some individuals may be exploited in any given society for the sake of those with power" (266). Feminist scholars have long criticized Western medicine as a significant contributor to sexist ideologies (e.g., Delaney et al. 1988; Ehrenreich and English 1973).

In expanding Goffman's conceptualization of tribal stigma, I note that women with chronic STDs internalize a degree of social stigma that medical sociologists have not typically associated with individuals infected with easily hidden diseases. Rather, researchers have connected social stigma with those experiencing discrediting illnesses. In reference to individuals with Parkinson's disease, urinary or bowl incontinence, Charmaz (2000) found that "guilt and shame increase when chronically ill people view themselves as socially incompetent" (285). Women with chronic STDs do not exhibit public signs of bodily abomination, and yet they experience feelings of social incompetence in their failure to remain in the tribe of "good girls." Future research on the experiences of men and women with sexual/reproductive illnesses should continue to examine the potency of gender expectations on affected individuals' experiences of stigma and identity, especially in matters of tribal stigma and social identity crises.

Morality and Medicine

The women's diagnostic and treatment narratives highlight the micro-level effects (e.g., patients' satisfaction and emotional distress/comfort) of our society having constructed certain types of patients as immoral, as well as the public health implications of compliance when morality mixes with medicine. Attitudes, beliefs, and behaviors that reinforce ideas that certain patients are immoral pose both individual-level and public health dilemmas.

Beyond sexual health, social mores shape health policy and social attitudes when diagnoses create patients who are judged according to the moral culpability of their condition. Examples of other "immoral patients" include alcoholics, drug addicts, smokers, and obese individuals. Gaussot (1998) studied the social construction of "good drinking" and found that individuals either viewed alcoholism as a disease, a sign of creativity, or proof of social and moral failure. Smyth's (1998) examination of the socio-historical understanding of the female alcoholic found that social texts contributed to the conception of alcoholic women as impoverished, neglectful of their children, and promiscuous. This "moral outcast" model of the alcoholic was found to promote secrecy and denial.

Drug users have also been found to employ the strategy of denial as a way to cope with a stigmatizing diagnosis. A study of injection drug users documented that they experienced an internal contradiction between their self-concepts as responsible and careful injectors and their admitted behaviors of high-risk borrowing and lending of injecting paraphernalia (Plumridge and Chetwynd 1998). These researchers found that this identity contradiction was resolved by producing discourses of exoneration that fit the moral implications of the different risk behaviors. However, the drug users put more energy towards and were more effective at shielding themselves from moral stigma than at reducing high-risk behaviors.

A similar lack of medical compliance has been found among individuals diagnosed as obese. "If the fitness 'revolution' was driven by scientific findings about risk and behavior, it also took on a powerful moral and prescriptive dimension" (Brandt 1997, 67). An interview study of obese individuals found that all had been subjected to "contemptuous" treatment from their doctors, and that the resulting "fear of humiliation prevents [them] from seeking health care" (Joanisse 1999, 14). If our society wants to develop effective treatment programs for illnesses, such as STDs, substance addiction, and obesity, then we would have to change, not only the judgmental attitudes of medical practitioners, but also the larger social messages that these conditions are "deserved" and brought on by "bad" behavior. Brandt (1997, 68) cautioned that deviant health behaviors "such as cigarette smoking are socio-cultural phenomena, not merely individual or necessarily rational choices." Therefore, the moral condemnation of a health condition that results from such behaviors is simplistic and inappropriate.

Stigma Management and Deviant Identity Formation

The women with STDs went through an emotionally difficult process, testing out stigma management strategies, trying to control the impact of STDs on both their self-concepts and on their relationships with others. In keeping with Cooley's "looking glass self" (1902/1964), the women I studied derived their sexual selves from the imagined and real reactions of others. Unable to immunize themselves from the physical wrath of disease, they focused on mediating potentially harmful impacts of STDs on their sexual self-concepts and on their intimate relationships. They accomplished this, via stigma denial, stigma transference, and stigma acceptance.

One model of deviant identity formation treats the process as involving three distinct, linear stages: *Primary, secondary* (Lemert 1967) and *tertiary deviance* (Kitsuse 1980). The women began the move into primary deviance when they engaged in the initial act of deviance—contraction of a sexually transmitted disease. However, the actual moment of STD transmission was imperceptible and did not result in a deviant label. Rather, in private interactions, medical practitioners named the deviance, via STD diagnoses, thus completing the women's transitions into primary deviance.

Movement into secondary deviance began as the women contemplated how they would manage the stigma of sexual disease in their "real" lives, beyond the sterile doors of examination rooms. As the women made choices about which stigma management strategies to use, they grappled with the ramifications of internalizing this new label. Choosing passing and covering techniques meant that they could remain in denial and put off internalizing a negative view of themselves. When they deflected the stigma onto others, via stigma transference, the women glimpsed the severity of STD stigma as reflected in the presumed sexual selves of real and imaginary others. Finally, the women's disclosures confirmed realities of having spoiled sexual selves.

For the women I studied, the stigma penetrated only the portions of their self-concepts that addressed sexuality. They were forced to reconcile new, "dirty" sexual self-concepts with their prior self-conceptions of unspoiled sexual health. However, all of them succeeded in compartmentalizing the deviant identity of being sexually diseased, relegating this deviant label to their sexual selves. They never completed transitions to secondary deviance, in which deviant identity becomes fully integrated into one's core self-concept (Lemert 1967). Unlike other medically deviant groups studied by ethnographers (Herman 1993, Karp 1992, Sandstrom 1990), the women in this study learned to accept a tainted sexual self, but did not internalize a deviant identity that spoiled their entire self-concept.

The data highlight the limitations of this three-stage model for explaining the process of deviant identity development for women with STDs. The fragmented nature of the women's movement into secondary deviance stems from the situational nature of genital herpes and/or HPV. Unlike diagnoses of HIV/AIDS—which carry the threat of life-changing illness, death, and contagion beyond the scope of sexual behaviors—chronic STD stigma lends itself to compartmentalization. The women were able to hide their shame, guilt, and fear (of further health complications, of contaminating others, of rejection, etc.) in the sexual part of their self-concepts. They recognized that this did not have to affect their overarching identities. Medically speaking, an STD need only affect the decisions and interactions connected with sexual and reproductive behavior. If the impact of the infections on their sex lives ever became too emotionally painful, the women could decide to distance themselves from sexual roles, choosing temporary or permanent celibacy.

Narrative Model of Self as a Stigma Management Strategy

A "narrative metaphor" for the self (Hermans 1996) views the self as multi-voiced. Historically, James (1890/1902) and Mead (1934) discussed the distinctions between the objective ("I") and subjective ("Me") selves. While the subjective self engages in self-reflexivity to negotiate an identity, information obtained by interacting with others continues to shape the objective self. In this way, the externally constructed self mediates internal conversations about identity. During these dialogues between the "I" and the "me," one's negotiated identities become incorporated into the self-concept.

James (1890/1902) posited the distinction between "I" and "me." However, Mancuso and Sarbin (1983/1986) posited an interpretation of James (1890/1902) and Mead (1934) that frames the I-Me distinction as a narrative of the self. From a narrative perspective, the "I" is the author of the story about "Me," the protagonist of the story being constructed about the self. The ability to construct such a narrative came from the I's ability to reinvent the past, hypothesize the future, and describe herself/himself as the actor (Crites 1986). In this way, the construction of self-narratives becomes the means by which individuals organize experiences, behaviors, and their accounts of these events (Sarbin 1986).

The narrative model of the self proposes that personal myths create the self and become "the stories we live by" (McAdams 1996, 266). I argue that we seek to understand the significance of the stories we choose *not* to live by. Personal STD "stories" are rarely told in American mass culture. McAdams (1996, 22) contended that "carrying on affairs in secret"—maintaining a discreditable stigma—is a way to keep stigmatizing stories "from occupying center stage" in people's personal myths. However, these data suggest that individuals manage identity transformations, especially transformations into deviant identities, by constructing and sharing self-narratives via disclosure interactions. While the women did not maintain secrecy, they did keep their STD stories from occupying "center stage."

When the distasteful or spoiled self can be contained to the private sphere (such as the sex life), the "I" employs stigma management strategies that protect the core self from the spoiled part of the self. To accomplish this, the "I" authors a *peripheral* narrative about the deviant aspect of the "Me." Disclosures are the telling of this peripheral narrative. This type of narrative is connected, yet fails to contaminate, the "core" narrative, in which the "Me," as protagonist, is insulated from the stigma contained in the peripheral narrative.

The incompleteness of the women's transitions into secondary deviance is explained by their choice to incorporate the stigma into a peripheral, rather than core self-narrative. Although this strategy enables them to protect their core self-narrative from stigma, the women face challenges in maintaining this compartmentalization. While celibacy is an obvious aid in utilizing this stigma management strategy (four participants were celibate at the times of their interviews), the norm of sexual activity repeatedly makes the sexual self a salient part of women's self-concepts. In modern American culture, "heterosexual activity is seen not only as desirable, but also as necessary for a 'normal' healthy life, [and] the pressures on women to marry or cohabit with a man, with all the consequent forms of servicing, are increased" (Walby 1990, 127).[4]

In many ways, the creation of a deviant peripheral self-narrative may be the ultimate stigma management strategy. The apparent effectiveness of this particular stigma management strategy might appeal to all individuals who struggle with deviant stigma. The rarity of its use is explained by the organizational complexity of those who share a particular deviant stigma. The existence of a deviant subculture promotes internalization of a deviant label (secondary deviance) by implying membership requirements: Acceptance of deviant norms, values, social support, etc. (Best and Luckenbill 1980). Deviant subcultures also allow for the existence of collective stigma management groups that may encourage individuals to move into tertiary deviance and embrace their deviant identities (Kitsuse 1980). The inclusion of stigmatized individuals into deviant subcultures exposes them to others, who have rewritten their core self-narratives to reflect their deviant identities. Such groups function to remove the negative connotation of the deviance by offering inclusion to their deviant circles (Lemert 1951). However, micro-level interactions between deviant individuals and collective stigma management groups encourage the incorporation of the stigmatized label into core self-narratives.

The data on how women manage the stigma of chronic STDs have implications for the study of isolated deviants and the study of self-transformation of deviants in general. They illuminate the role of isolation in protecting a core self-narrative from stigma. Individuals, such as women with STDs, remain loners because their deviant labels do not provide them with membership to deviant subcultures (Lowery and Wetli 1982) and, possibly, to collective stigma management groups. When society constructs a type of deviance as "loner," affected individuals do not need to enter complete secondary deviance and internalize the deviant label into their core self-narrative. Isolated in their experience of this stigma, these individuals have greater flexibility in their decision to rewrite their deviant transformations into either core or peripheral self-narratives. Further research on loner deviants would be helpful in testing the efficacy of peripheral self-narratives for managing stigma.

Overall, I hope that *Damaged Goods* adds to our knowledge of how individuals, especially women, are impacted by living with incurable sexually transmitted diseases. By examining how these women made sense of their illness experiences, I aim to expand sociological interpretations of sexual stories and illness narratives and provide an original contribution to studies, which focus on the intersections of sex, gender, stigma, and chronic illness.

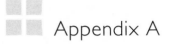

Appendix A

Gaining Entrée—An Auto-Ethnographic Foundation

Some experiences are private and so painful that it takes years before one can talk openly about them. Four years after I was diagnosed and treated for a cervical HPV infection, I decided to disclose to friends and colleagues, while in graduate school. Part of my commitment to managing my own sexual health status was to become educated and, then, to help educate others: I trained first as a peer educator and, ultimately, became employed as a professional sexual health educator. I also began to invest my activist and academic energies into helping others who found themselves enmeshed in a similar STD crisis.

My STD experiences gave me the standpoint of an "auto-ethnographer" (Hayano 1979), in that I shared the same "master status" (Hughes 1945) as those I studied. I entered the research setting in the role of "complete member" (Adler and Adler 1987) and, in many ways, related to participants as their "status equal." Though I had more education and professional experience with STDs than most of my participants, I shared many of the same experiences and feelings associated with having a chronic STD. My lived experiences with HPV served as a primary motivation for conducting this research and, undoubtedly, shaped my initial conceptualizations for analyzing the data. As an ethnographer, my eyes, ears, and brain were the tools for data collection and analysis. A few weeks after completing my final interview for this study, I wrote down my own STD illness narrative. I applied the conceptual categories and analyzed my story, as I had the other participants'. While I believe that I could not have conducted this study without an insider's perspective, I view my experiences with STDs as a salient factor in explaining how I created trust and rapport with participants, as a potential influence on my methodology, and a possible bias affecting my analysis of the data.

My Auto-ethnography

The story told at the beginning of this book is the beginning of my own story. What follows is the complete story of my STD experience, including an auto-ethnographic analysis of how my experiences fit with the *Six Stages of Sexual-Self Transformation* that I developed for this research. My greatest challenge in writing up the data came, not from having to synthesize the experiences of my participants, but from having to produce and reflect on the content of my auto-ethnography. Knowing early on in my study that methodological honesty required the telling of my story, I had felt prepared to write this piece. However, the process of putting into words what had, until that point, been carefully compartmentalized within my sexual self proved to be more painful than I had anticipated. Comfortable in my present-day skin of being a sexual health researcher and educator, I dreaded dismantling my persona of expertise and owning the vulnerable, scared, young woman I had been. Reflecting on my past helped me to locate myself as a researcher on the "same critical plane as the overt subject matter" (Harding 1987, 8). Ultimately, I hope that my analytical writings on the participants' illness narratives retained the authenticity that I strove to reveal in my auto-ethnography.

My Story

As a 20-year-old undergraduate, I received a phone call from my ex-boyfriend. He nervously told me that he had just been diagnosed with genital warts and was in the process of having them "frozen off" with liquid nitrogen. He explained that he called because there was a chance that he might have had *this* when we had last *been together*. He added that he was not sure if I was at risk because he had not noticed symptoms until recently. I quickly thanked him for calling, hung up the phone, and sat in stunned silence.

I thought to myself: *How could this have happened to me? I'm not a slut: I've only had sex with three guys and always used condoms. I talked with both my ex boyfriends and current boyfriend before we ever had se—they told me about their sexual histories and sexual health. These guys had all tested negative for HIV, so they were "safe"—healthy and trustworthy—right? My high-school sex education focused on HIV/AIDS, so I've only been worried about fluids being transmitted. Is it possible to get a disease even when you're using condoms?*

A series of scary questions ran through my mind. *Do I have warts, too? How could I, when my last annual gynecological exam was less than six*

*months ago, and my Pap smear results were normal? Wouldn't my doctor
have noticed if I had warts? Could I have warts that are so tiny I've never
noticed them? Have I already infected my current boyfriend?* With no answers to any of these questions, one horrific image appeared in my mind with
unsettling clarity: Inspired by the one film about other sexually transmitted
diseases (STDs), which was shown in my high-school health class, I envisioned my vulva sprouting cauliflower-like growths, more and more fleshy
warts, ultimately covering my genitals inside and out. This image brought me
to tears. As I began to cry, I wondered: *Will any guy ever want me? Will I
ever get married or be able to have a healthy baby?*

In a rash state of mind, the next call I made was to my current boyfriend.
Feeling that he was sure to dump me after hearing what I had to say, I decided
to be preemptive. In an eerily calm tone, I told him that I had just found out I
had been exposed to and, in all likelihood, contracted genital warts. I said that
I was calling him so that he could get tested and to say that I was very sorry to
have given him an STD. Before he could digest and react to the news, I informed him that I would be going to the doctor next week and would call him
once I had definite results. But, right now, I needed some time to process this
on my own, so it was best for us not to see each other until I knew what was
going on. Before he had a chance to respond, I apologized again and said
"goodbye."

At my gynecology appointment, the nurse practitioner did a Pap smear
and a visual inspection, telling me that she could see no evidence of genital
warts, but would know more in a week, once she had the results of my Pap
smear. When I got home, I called up my ex-boyfriend to tell him about my appointment and ended up asking to meet with him that night. By this time,
even in the absence of a diagnosis, I was beginning to feel like no man would
ever want to be with me sexually for fear of the risk. Sitting face to face with
my ex, I not only saw a man whom I still loved, but also the one person who
could truly empathize with my condition, possibly the one man who would not
blame or condemn me for it because he had likely given it to me. That night,
we began the discussion that would ultimately lead to me breaking up with my
current boyfriend and getting back together with my ex.

A few days later, my practitioner called with the results of my Pap smear:
Abnormal with evidence of "condyloma plana." She referred me to a gynecologist who would perform a "colposcopy" and "biopsy the affected tissue" to
confirm the severity of my "HPV infection." Confused by her medical terminology, I asked what all of the terms meant. She explained that "condyloma
plana" refers to flat lesions, invisible to the naked eye, of which evidence had
been found in her scraping of my cervical tissue. A colposcopy was a diagnostic procedure, whereby the doctor would apply an acetic acid (white vinegar)
solution to my external and internal genitals and use a colposcope, a high-power
microscope, to search for HPV-infected cells. Infected cells would react to the
acetic acid by turning white. If any of these "white" cells were found, the

doctor would perform *punch* biopsies, use an instrument similar to a cookie cutter to remove pieces of the white areas and send these samples off to the lab to be tested for HPV. Confused that she had not used the term "genital warts," I asked if I had them. She replied that what I had was evidence of HPV, human papillomavirus—the virus that causes genital warts. I did not appear to have any visible warts, only the viral lesions on my cervix, but that I might yet develop genital warts.

Feeling more confused than before, I began a process of self-education that took me from the campus women's resource center, to the student health center, to the library. My goal was to find out everything I could about HPV and genital warts. What are the specific diagnostic tests? How do they treat cervical versus external infections? How exactly is the virus transmitted? Finally, and most importantly, is there a cure?

My findings did more to fuel my anxieties than to quiet my fears. I discovered that there are more than 70 types of HPV, approximately 20 viral types infect genital tissue: Of those, 13 have been linked by medical researchers to cervical, vaginal, penile, and anal cancer (Keller et al.1995). I found out that my medical insurance would pay for a lab to determine if I had HPV, but would not cover viral-typing to determine if I was at higher risk for cervical cancer. My nurse practitioner assured me that it really was not worth the extra expense because the treatment plan would be the same in any case: The goal of any treatment was to kill and remove as much of the HPV-infected tissue as possible.[i] However, I learned that the disease was considered chronic and incurable because there could never be absolute assurance that every, single HPV-infected cell had been removed.

I discovered that treatments for mild cases of external warts included topical applications of acid or liquid nitrogen, in addition to less effective creams and ointments. Moderate cervical cases required cryosurgery: The application of liquid nitrogen directly to the cervix that killed the tissue it touched. Severe cases of external and cervical HPV could be treated via laser: Slicing off and simultaneously cauterizing the tissue. Deep infections of the cervix that bordered on cancer required the use of loop electrocautery excision procedure (LEEP) or cold knife conization. Both of these options removed large portions of the infected cervix, while leaving as much as possible, so that the cervix might ultimately regenerate to the thickness required to bear the weight of a growing fetus. Finally, if HPV had progressed to cervical cancer, it was possible that the entire cervix and uterus would have to be removed: Medically this is called a *simple* hysterectomy because the ovaries are left.

The idea that I might be facing the end of my fertility shattered the core of my sexual self. While I had spent the last three and a half years trying very

---

[i]"HPV targets the basal layer of the epidermis or mucosa" (Keller et al.1995, 351).

hard *not* to get pregnant, I had always assumed that I *could* and *would* get pregnant someday. The ability to conceive a child was a given in my pre-HPV world. The only questions had been when and with whom? Admittedly in a pessimistic mindset, I imagined ten years into the future, being married to a wonderful man, and feeling guilty and heartbroken that we could not have biological children together.

At this point, I decided to call my parents. I had always had a close relationship with both my mom and dad: For example, I had told them both about my first sexual experience, and my mom had accompanied me to my first gynecological exam. I was scared and deeply needed their reassurance that everything was going to be okay. My mom was the first to react after hearing what had happened. She was angry. In fact, it would not be an overstatement to say she was furious with my ex (then, newly current) boyfriend. While on the phone, I rehashed my hypothesis that he had contracted the HPV from a woman he had dated before getting back together with me the time prior. This woman he had dated had been older and was known to have "slept around" with a lot of guys. I remembered him having told me she was sterile, a seemingly strange fact for a woman only 27 years old. Now, as I talked with my parents, I shared my fears that perhaps she had been sterile because of severe cervical HPV infection. The idea that I, too, could become sterile from this disease made me hysterical and made my parents determined to help me receive the highest quality medical care.

The next step was to see the gynecologist. He brusquely explained the colposcopy procedure. Having been forewarned about punch biopsies, I asked whether he could provide any pain medication. Appearing confused by my request, he said he supposed I could have some Extra Strength Tylenol, but he claimed that no patient of his had ever seemed to need any medication for this procedure. I took him up on the offer and braced myself in the stirrups. The vinegar solution stung a little as he peered through the colposcope muttering to his nurse the location of each biopsy site before "punching" out a piece. He took samples not only from my cervix, for which I was prepared, but also from my labia. As he removed the labial samples, I again recalled my high-school health class slide of wart-covered genitalia. In a short time, he was done and told me that I should make an appointment to come back in two weeks, at which time he would be able to tell me what parts of me were infected with HPV and if I had cervical cancer.

Cancer. The word wrapped itself around my throat, making it hard to talk with the receptionist when I had to make the follow-up appointment. Cancer. I was only 20 years old, how could I have cancer? I did not smoke, never did drugs, and rarely drank. But, I had been sexually active, and obviously there was a punishment to be borne for this sin. How could I have been so stupid? Could even the most pleasurable sexual experience in the world be worth the worry and torment of the next two weeks?

My roommate drove me to the doctor's office for the fateful follow-up appointment. I had a feeling that whatever the results, I might not be in a condition to safely drive myself home. After checking in with the receptionist, she ushered us into a room with an examination table and a large, imposing canister of liquid nitrogen. Sitting, fully dressed, upon the paper-sheet-covered table, I looked at my roommate and began to cry. Before she could say anything, the gynecologist walked in and was clearly surprised to see an extra person in the room. Explaining that he was ready to perform cryosurgery on me today, he questioned why I was so upset.

At this point, I lost it—yelling at him and crying at the same time. He had not even bothered to tell me the lab results, to tell me which parts of my body were infected, let alone to sit me down and discuss treatment options. Shocked by my emotions, he said that the labial samples had come back negative but the cervical samples came back "positive and mild," so cryosurgery was the best option. Now on the verge of hyperventilating, I shouted at him: "This was supposed to be my diagnostic visit! You were supposed to sit me down in your office and talk things through with me!" I was irate and confused, unable to slow down my thoughts and process the information he had vaguely given to me. That particular day, I had my period and knew from my research that cryosurgery would have to wait. I angrily informed him that even after my period was over, he would not be the one to treat me. Then, I launched into an attack of his bedside manner: "Under no circumstances should you ever carelessly toss out the possibility of cancer to a patient and leave them to worry about it for two weeks! Especially when you're talking to a younger female patient who would likely be worried about her fertility—you should have the lab results to back up any talk of cancer!" With that said, I left his office, never to return.

During this stage, my family's socioeconomic status played an important role. That doctor had been the only local gynecologist covered under my parents' health insurance. After doing some research on gynecologists in the area, I found a specialty clinic that focused exclusively on women's health and featured only female gynecologists. My parents readily agreed to pay the extra costs, and my mother accompanied me to the consultation. After looking over my records and test results, the new gynecologist concurred that cryosurgery was the best choice, and then she explained exactly why it was best, and why other options were less optimal. At ease with her bedside manner and confident in her expertise, I scheduled the procedure.

The morning of the cryosurgery I was nervous but also excited to have the infected and contagious cells permanently removed from my body. This time, I was ready. My mom accompanied me to the appointment and stayed in the room during the procedure. Having taken some stronger pain medication, I did not expect to feel the trauma to my cervix. I learned quickly that this organ does not feel "normal" pain like one's external skin. Rather, the pain is beyond the worst menstrual cramps imaginable and seemed closer to what I had heard described by other women as labor contractions. However, in a short time the pain was over: The surface of my cervix was frozen, and I was sent home to rest.

For the next ten days, my frozen cervical cells sloughed off as a smelly, grayish sludge from my body. While I had been medically forbidden to have sexual intercourse for at least two weeks, I found myself in no rush. It was difficult to feel sexy when my vagina was draining, my labia were healing (from technically unnecessary biopsies), and my current sexual partner had sore spots of nitrogen burn on his penis from his own wart removals. I looked forward to the series of follow-up colposcopy procedures and Pap smears, hoping I would ultimately find out that the worst was over because the HPV would not reappear.

Fortunately, my cryosurgery was very successful. All of my follow-up exams returned results of "normal" Pap smears. However, having learned that it was still theoretically possible for me to have HPV infected cells, lurking beyond the range of the cervical surface that was scraped during a standard Pap smear, I made it a policy to always tell partners of my STD status. In addition to asking partners about their sexual health history, I also requested that they be thoroughly screened for STDs prior to us engaging in any "risky" behavior: My new definition of risky behaviors now included any genital skin-to-skin contact, so this meant even those who had always used latex/male condoms consistently and correctly could still have put themselves at risk for contracting HPV and or genital herpes infections.

Four years after cryosurgery, I was in a new relationship and wanted to know if I would be putting my current partner at risk for HPV, if I were to go on the pill and give up condoms. As a graduate student, I had joined the campus health center's sexual health peer education program and begun to collaborate on projects with the women's health clinic staff. Due to this growing level of trust and rapport, I felt comfortable being assertive during my annual gynecological exam and Pap smear, and I asked the nurse practitioner whether I might be able to schedule a colposcopy even though my Pap smear results would likely reveal nothing abnormal. This is not standard procedure, but I knew that this might be the only way for me to achieve the peace of mind needed to have unprotected contact with my current partner. Given my history with HPV and our friendship, she referred me to the gynecologist who understood that my goal was to determine if I still had any HPV-infected cells. The gynecologist thoroughly coated my internal and external genitals in the acetic acid solution. When one area of cervical cells did turn white, she took a biopsy of those cells: The biopsy results found no trace of HPV.

Finally, over eight years after the fateful phone call, I completed this research project and felt that I was reasonably whole and healthy again. Though, I must admit that whenever I feel or see any abnormality on my genital tissue (razor burn, ingrown hair, etc.) my first suspicion is always genital warts.

When I became pregnant in 2003, the fear renewed: Could the hormonal changes of pregnancy or strain of childbirth coax "theoretically possible" HPV-infected cells out of their dormant states and renew my cervical infection? Would my baby become infected during delivery? The answers to those questions, thankfully, were two resounding "No's"—I was fortunate to have a normal pregnancy and deliver a healthy, baby girl. Now, it is almost hard for me to believe the amount of stress and emotional pain I went through over a decade ago. Sadly, as a college professor who teaches courses on sexuality, deviance, and medical sociology, I am reminded by my students in the classroom and in private discussions every semester, that today's young women continue to experience the anxiety, pain, and crises that stem from being diagnosed with highly stigmatizing STDs.

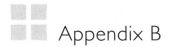 Appendix B

Research Methodology

My decision to focus my study on women was based on preliminary reading and informal discussions with sexual health practitioners and educators. The consensus was that women's experiences of STDs were different from those of men, in light of gender role expectations around sexual morality and behavior. I decided to focus on women with chronic/viral, non-HIV STDs, specifically genital herpes and HPV. Having talked with friends who had had curable (typically bacterial) STDs, I learned that their illness experiences were so brief and lacking in long-term effects that none felt there had been any lasting effects on their sexual selves. However, the friends of mine who had genital herpes and/or HPV infections had stories of illness experiences that were poignant and still relevant in their lives, as they continued to deal with new outbreaks, treatments, issues of disclosure with sexual partners, and concerns about their reproductive health.

While HIV is a chronic/viral STD, I ruled it out as a focus for several reasons. First, the physiological reality of this disease is far more serious than any other STD in contemporary times. In addition, the social dynamics of this epidemic are such that public awareness campaigns, activist organizations, and anti-AIDS forces have shaped a unique socio-medical context. Many researchers have conducted HIV/AIDS studies that span disciplines from the life sciences, to the social sciences, to communication studies and beyond. This is a highly saturated research area, and I believed I was in a unique position to contribute to a subject and group of people who had been largely neglected by scientists, scholars, and the media.

Evolution of the Research Design

While working as a sexual health educator, I began to question how infected women managed the various challenges of lifelong but manageable STD infections. Only a small percentage of STD-infected women attend organized support groups, the setting in which I initially hoped to conduct this research. My research methods evolved from overt participant-observation of an STD support group, to a survey that investigated women's attitudes about STDs, and finally into an in-depth interview study. Having experienced and heard first-hand accounts of problematic medical encounters, I was committed to utilizing qualitative methods as a way to shape a research project, such that it had a "critical focus on the institution of medicine" (Charmaz and Olesen 1997, 453). While the qualitative research paradigm advocates studying social phenomena within social settings, it is not always possible to find a physical setting in which a particular social group congregates. Public health statistics on genital herpes and HPV assured me that there were large numbers of women and men living with these diseases. However, there were no formal or informal STD support groups in my area.

Sampling Methods

My first hurdle was to obtain approval from the university's Human Research Committee. Their main concern was the participants' confidentiality. As individuals' medical records of STD diagnoses and treatment are confidential, I was not allowed to directly recruit participants. Rather, participants had to approach me, usually after hearing me present on sexual health, seeing my flyers, or hearing about my research from other participants. The criteria for participation included being at least eighteen years of age, having been diagnosed with genital herpes and/or HPV, and a willingness to talk about personal and interpersonal effects of the illness.

Once interview participants contacted me, I gained entrée and acceptance via my statuses as a sexual health educator and a complete member. As has been the case with many studies of individuals living with HIV/AIDS (Cranson and Caron 1998; Grove et al.1997; Sandstrom 1996), I employed a convenience sampling method because of the sensitive nature of the topic—random sampling of the population was not possible. I ended interviews with requests that, if they felt comfortable, they might tell appropriate friends about my research. In this way, I utilized snowball sampling (Biernacki and Waldorf 1981) to generate interviews. In keeping with grounded theory, my goal was to sample for theory construction, rather than for representativeness (Charmaz 1995).

All forty-three participants identified themselves as having been diagnosed with genital herpes and/or HPV. In all, eleven of the women were diagnosed with genital herpes infections, and thirty-two with HPV infections. Of these forty-three women, three had been diagnosed with both genital herpes and HPV. The women with HPV diagnoses included nineteen who had been diagnosed with cervical lesions, eight with external genital warts, and five with both cervical and external HPV infections. Appendix C (pages 210–211) charts several demographic characteristics of these participants.

For purposes of categorization, I relied on each participant's self-stated identity of their demographic descriptors. The women ranged in age from 19 to 56. The women I interviewed were consistent with the demographics of the Rocky Mountain community. However, the sample was not necessarily representative of the population of women in the United States living with herpes and/or HPV, as it skewed toward a high percentage of white women with higher socioeconomic statuses and above-average educational attainment. However, women's health researchers have noted that "the urban minority poor" were "the population most likely to be studied by researchers working on STDs" and recommended, "A broader range of populations should be studied" (Leonardo and Chrisler 1992, 13).

As such, my sample demographically represented an atypical population for STD research. Thirty-eight of the women were Caucasian (including those who self-identified as Jewish, Greek, and Persian); three were Latino, one was African American, and one was Native American. Socioeconomically, they ranged from working-class (9) to upper-class (1), with the majority identifying as lower-middle (5), middle (18) or upper-middle (10) class. The respondents represented a wide variety of religious upbringings and current practices including, Buddhists, Christians, Jews, Muslims, Pagans, Protestants, and Southern Baptists. The largest religious representation was Catholic (12), although fourteen identified as having been raised with no religion, with nineteen identifying as currently non-religious. In the matter of sexual identity, the majority (37) identified as heterosexual, while five identified as being bisexual, and one identified as a lesbian.

Data Collection

My research was conducted over a four-year period (1997–2000). I developed a semi-structured interview schedule that covered the following topics:

- Demographic data
- Early sexual education experiences (both formal and informal)
- Memories of rumors, gossip, or first-hand experiences with girls or women who were considered promiscuous
- Negotiating sexual relationships (including nonconsensual sex)
- Later sexual health education experiences
- Becoming infected
- Being diagnosed
- Receiving treatments
- Advice for sexual health practitioners
- Advice for young women

At appropriate points throughout the interview, I inquired as to how they remembered feeling about themselves as sexual beings: As children, adolescents, teenagers, pre-STD infection, at diagnosis, during treatments, etc. The interview gave each woman the opportunity to tell me, in her own words, what had been, and continued to be, important to her about specific sexual health issues, and how having a chronic STD was affecting her life.

I conducted the interviews in private locations of the participants' preferences. The interviews lasted from forty-five minutes to two and-a-half hours and were tape recorded with the permission of the participants. To ensure confidentiality, I had participants read and sign informed consent forms that specified I would be using pseudonyms and destroying all evidence (cassettes, master code lists, etc.) at the conclusion of the study, so that they could not be linked to having participated.

I constructed my research methods to reflect a reciprocal intention. During the interviews, I would offer my empathy and share appropriate pieces of my own story to create a feeling of mutual vulnerability. At the conclusion of interviews, I would offer my support and resources as a sexual health educator. When appropriate, I offered to provide sexual health information and resources, either in the form of health education materials or referrals to resources.

While methodologists have criticized single interviews for providing a glimpse, rather than the whole story, the sensitivity of the subject matter (participation was often dependent upon only having to talk once) and transitory nature of the sample (approximately 75 percent were undergraduate or graduate college students) made it improbable for me to conduct follow-up interviews with participants. Inherent in the inability to conduct follow-up interviews with all participants, I was also unable to receive input on my final analysis from all participants. However, six participants who remained in contact with me after being interviewed were given the opportunity to critique portions of the analytical product.

Many researchers have gone against traditional methods of interviewing that emphasize distance, instead answering participants' questions, providing important educational information, and maintaining friendships with participants long after studies reached completion (Nielson 1990). This style of ethnography favors semi-structured or unstructured interviewing because it "produces non-standardized information that allows researchers to make full use of differences among people" (Reinharz 1990, 19). During the interviews, I used researcher self-disclosure to create and maintain rapport, as have other researchers of illness who are complete members. Fundamentally, "uncertainty is made livable through dialogue" (Frank 1997, 29), and I tried to maintain a feeling of a mutual conversation, rather than interacting as a non-emotive interviewer. I also included self-reflexive reporting of the interview process as part of the transcribed data that I analyzed (Reinharz 1990).

In keeping with Oakley's (1981) feminist critique of interview methodology, I did not rule out answering questions asked by participants. Rather, I incorporated an educational stance and expressed my willingness to answer any questions about sexual health (modes of transmission, diagnostic procedures, treatment options, etc.) after the conclusion of our "official" interview. In many cases, I worked hard to maintain my composure when a participant related incorrect information, including that which had been delivered to them by medical practitioners. At the conclusion of such interviews, I would mention that I had made some notes of possible misinformation and ask if they would like me to discuss and correct the inaccuracies. All of the participants who had been misinformed did ask for accurate updates. While some found out "good news," most who had been misinformed felt disheartened by news that their infections were more contagious, more chronic, or might require additional treatments.

In all, I conducted forty-three conversational, semi-structured interviews with consensual participants. The end sample size is partially the result of sampling limitations. Given ethical restrictions on participant recruitment, I could not obtain a list of all women in the geographic area who fit my study's criteria in order to generate a random sample. With this limitation, and my interest in building theory, theoretical sampling became my goal. As I will elaborate on in the following section, the end sample size also represents a point of saturation with reference to theoretical themes, coding categories and sub-categories.

Data Analysis

Interviews were transcribed in their entirety. I analyzed the data according to the principles of grounded theory, using constant comparative methods (Glaser and Strauss 1967; Glaser 1978) to adjust analytical categories to fit emerging theoretical concepts. In keeping with this approach, I began to analyze transcribed data during the first months of interviewing, identifying primary themes and concepts that emerged from participants' narratives. As data patterns reappeared, I verified some categories and discarded others.

Initially, I used introspection (Ellis 1991) to hypothesize stages of how women's sexual-self concepts were impacted by being diagnosed and treated for chronic STDs. With each interview, I clustered participants' experiences around particular stages to assess the validity of my initial model. The six stages of sexual-self transformation emerged from the data as follows: Sexual invincibility, STD suspicion, diagnostic crisis, stigma management, healing/treatment, and reintegration. I developed this stage analysis of the transformative effects of STDs on women's sexual selves to better understand their lived illness experiences and narratives. I agree with Frank (1997) that, "the narrative [focus] is fundamentally about accepting the ill person's need to sustain a sense of authenticity of her experience" (Frank 1997:28). My analytical goals were ultimately to achieve high construct validity and authenticity.

I then looked through transcriptions of the interviews for illustrations of the stages, examining each example to further check the validity of my conceptualizations. As certain stages emerged, I began to ask about them more specifically in interviews, checking for the boundaries and variations as applied concepts. I also searched for connections between different stages and sub-components, searching to understand how these conceptualizations interacted with each other. When particular stages emerged as more dominant themes in interviews, I centered my thinking around them as key analytical concepts. The resulting evolutionary analysis was what Wiseman (1970) called a "total pattern," a sequence of events that held true for the group studied. During the process of data collection and analysis, my goal was to remain connected to the meanings shared by the women interviewed, while constructing a theoretical framework that would sociologically represent their meanings within a symbolic interactionist perspective. I chose symbolic interactionism as my guiding analytical framework because it focuses on the self and human experience as socially constructed, via interactive processes. I followed this plan of data collection and analysis to maximize the validity of my findings.

When I had interviewed approximately thirty women, I reached a point of initial saturation: The emerging conceptual categories of my analysis had begun to "gel." Each new interview served to confirm rather than to create new categories. However, in acknowledgement of the self-selection bias of my sample and lack of representativeness with regards to race/ethnicity, class, age, and sexual identity, I continued to accept new invitations to interview. My hope was to expand the diversity of my sample as much as possible and further test the construct validity of my analytical coding. A few of the new interviews allowed me to refine coding categories, and with the conclusion of my forty-third interview, I reached the point of saturation. That is not to say that a similar study with ethical and practical allowances to organize a larger and randomly selected sample might not reach different analytical conclusions.

Methodological Challenges

During the course of this project, I faced challenges in research design, data collection, data analysis, and writing that were uniquely tied to the subject of STDs. As detailed earlier, my research design underwent several revisions until it culminated in an interview study. Lacking the opportunity for participant-observation, I had to rely on the veracity of participants' self-reporting. This was particularly pertinent with regards to the women's descriptions of medical encounters. However, I reconciled that a "fly on the wall approach" to observing patient encounters was completely unethical, and

I was more intrigued by the women's recollections of these events as meaningful to understanding their personal experiences of illness. For example, if a woman recalled being spoken to harshly by a judgmental practitioner, then her construction of that interaction was more significant towards understanding her illness narrative than my knowing the objective tone and content of that practitioner's words.

In the arena of data collection, I had anticipated difficulties gaining participants' respect and trust in the format of a one-time interview. However, this did not prove to be a problem. My background as a professional sexual health educator served to legitimate my intentions. In addition, my complete membership role and disclosure of my STD status strengthened participants' views of me as a researcher, with integrity and commitment to using their stories to help the cause of STD education, support, and treatment. The challenge arose when my role as researcher conflicted with my role as health educator. As explained earlier in this chapter, many of the women arrived at their interviews with incorrect and incomplete information about their diagnosis, prognosis, and/or treatment options. I felt obligated to remain in the researcher role until the interview's conclusion when I could, with the participant's permission, switch into educator mode. I felt it was my ethical obligation to provide them with as much accurate information as possible (e.g., brochures, pamphlets, newsletters from creditable national health agencies), so that they could go forward from the interview with a knowledge base that could inform their future decisions.

At the stage of data analysis, challenges became manifest in the area of timing. Recruitment for the study was difficult and unpredictable: some months I would be contacted by four women, other months zero. Following the guidelines of grounded theory and constant comparative analysis required that I put my analysis on hold during the "dry spells" so that I did not rush to conclusions that might be proven invalid with the next batch of interviews. My patience was tested, as I held off on confirming my analytical categories and sub-components until I felt I had at least reached a point of initial saturation: Approximately twenty-eight interviews and two years into the study.

My overarching goal in this study was to specify the different ways in which women are impacted by incurable sexually transmitted diseases. My aim was to consider how social contexts and personal experiences gave meaning to the different stages of their illnesses. Utilizing in-depth, semi-structured interviews and narrative analysis, I was able to generate theories and explore the complex intersections of illness stigma and identity formation. I was also able to examine the impact of cultural constructions of femininity and sexual morality, focusing on the ways in which intrapersonal conceptualizations of self and interpersonal constructions of status mediate women's experiences of these diseases. Having analyzed these interviews, I hope that I have provided readers with a complex and nuanced view of what it means to be women living with genital herpes and HPV infections in the U.S. today.

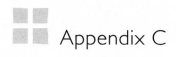

Appendix C

DEMOGRAPHIC CHARACTERISTICS OF PARTICIPANTS[1]

Pseudonym	Age	HSV?	HPV?	Racial/Ethnic Group	Social Class	Relationship Status	Children	Sexual Orientation
Amelia	26	No	Yes	White	Middle class	Living w/ long-term partner	None	Heterosexual
Anne	28	Yes	No	White	Lower-middle class	Living w/ long-term partner	None	Bisexual
Ashley	21	No	Yes	White	Upper middle class	Single/Dating	None	Heterosexual
Caprice	35	No	Yes	White	Working class	Single/Dating	None	Bisexual
Chris	40	Yes	No	White	Middle class	Single/Dating	None	Heterosexual
Cleo	31	No	Yes	White	Middle class	Married	1	Heterosexual
Deborah	32	No	Yes	White	Upper middle class	Single/Dating	None	Heterosexual
Diana	45	Yes	Yes	African-American	Upper middle class	Single/Dating	None	Heterosexual
Elle	32	Yes	No	White	Working class	Single/Dating	None	Bisexual
Francine	43	Yes	Yes	White	Middle class	Married	1	Heterosexual
Gita	23	No	Yes	Persian-American	Middle class	Single/Dating	None	Heterosexual
Gloria	47	Yes	Yes	Chicana	Working-class	Widowed/Dating	3	Heterosexual
Haley	22	No	Yes	White	Upper middle class	Single/Dating	None	Heterosexual
Heidi	31	No	Yes	White	Working class	Single/Dating	None	Heterosexual
Helena	31	No	Yes	Greek-American	Middle class	Single/Dating	None	Heterosexual
Hillary	22	No	Yes	White	Middle class	Single/Celibate	None	Heterosexual
Ingrid	23	No	Yes	White	Middle class	Single/Dating	None	Heterosexual
Janine	50	Yes	No	White	Middle class	Single/Dating	None	Heterosexual
Jasmine	20	No	Yes	White	Upper class	Single/Dating	None	Heterosexual
Jenny	18	No	Yes	White	Upper middle class	Single/Dating	None	Heterosexual

Name			Age	Race/ethnicity	Social class	Relationship status	Children	Sexual orientation
Julia	No	Yes	50	White	Middle class	Divorced/Celibate	None	Lesbian
Kayla	Yes	No	22	White	Working class	Engaged	None	Heterosexual
Kelly	Yes	No	31	White	Middle class	Married	None	Heterosexual
Lily	Yes	No	40	White	Middle class	Single/Dating	1	Heterosexual
Lola	Yes	No	30	White	Lower middle class	Single/Dating	None	Heterosexual
Louise	Yes	No	28	White	Middle class	Single/Not dating	None	Heterosexual
Marissa	Yes	No	31	Hispanic	Lower middle class	Single/Celibate	None	Heterosexual
Mary	Yes	No	51	White	Lower middle class	Divorced/Celibate	None	Heterosexual
Molly	Yes	No	43	White	Middle class	Married	3	Heterosexual
Monica	Yes	No	21	White	Middle class	Single/Dating	None	Heterosexual
Natasha	Yes	No	20	White	Middle class	Single/Dating	None	Heterosexual
Pam	Yes	No	42	White	Working class	Married	None	Heterosexual
Rebecca	No	Yes	56	White	Upper middle class	Married	None	Heterosexual
Rhonda	No	Yes	23	Hispanic (Cuban-American)	Working class	Single/Dating	None	Heterosexual
Robin	Yes	No	21	White	Upper middle class	Single/Dating	None	Heterosexual
Sam	Yes	No	34	White	Working class	Single/Dating	None	Heterosexual
Sandy	Yes	No	21	White	Middle class	Single/Not dating	None	Heterosexual
Sarah	Yes	No	24	White/Jewish	Upper middleclass	Living w/ long-term partner	None	Heterosexual
Sierra	Yes	No	23	White	Middle class	Single/Dating	None	Heterosexual
Summer	Yes	No	20	Native American	Lower-Middle class	Single/Dating	None	Bisexual
Tanya	No	Yes	27	White	Upper middle class	Single/Dating	None	Heterosexual
Tasha	Yes	No	30	White	Middle class	Single/Dating	None	Bisexual
Violet	Yes	No	35	White	Upper middle class	Single/Dating	None	Heterosexual

1 All characteristics were true of the participant at the time of the interview. Both race/ethnicity and social class reflect how the participant identified themselves when asked at the interview.

Notes

Chapter 1: Mixing Morality with Medicine

1. While some organizations, such as *Planned Parenthood*, prefer the term "STI" ("sexually transmitted infection"), I opted to employ the term "STD," in that it remains the standard nomenclature for the *Centers for Disease Control*.

2. Certain types of HPV may cause *respiratory papillomatosis*, lesions in the larynx and trachea, in infants of infected mothers (Centers for Disease Control 1999).

3. "There are about 30 variants of the virus that commonly infect men and women" (Brody 2007).

4. While, in many cases, HPV infections are likely to be resolved by individuals' immune systems "without clinical consequence" (Friedman and Shepeard 2007, 11), many cases do require treatment. Even after treatment, there is always the possibility that cervical lesions and/or genital warts could return because the virus may still be present.

5. Genital HPV and HSV infections are usually transmitted via penetrative intercourse (vaginal or anal), although, transmission by non-penetrative genital contact and oral-genital transmission has also been reported.

6. While a woman's cervical cells can be tested for HPV, there is no comparable test for other genital tissue, which leaves women with non-cervical HPV and all men unable to be tested for HPV.

7. HSV, in pregnant women, can cause fatal neonatal infections (Kimberlin 2004).

8. Dinh and Benoit (2007) define a prophylactic vaccine: "In contrast to treating established HPV infection using a vaccine, primary prevention of

HPV infection and the development of HPV-related diseases is achieved by immunizing those at risk for HPV" (481).

9. Abstinence from sexual behaviors that allow for skin-to-skin contact is the safest practice, but vaccinated females should also limit their number of sexual partners, practice monogamy, and use latex or polyurethane barriers with sexual partners.

10. Please see Appendix A for my auto-ethnography.

Chapter 2: Sexual Invincibility

1. "The effectiveness of condoms to prevent transmission is under debate" (Keller et al.1995:354): Vulvar and scrotal tissue infected with HPV or herpes are not covered by condoms, so the skin-to-skin contact necessary for viral transmission can occur even with the correct and consistent use of latex condoms. However, researchers still contend that condom usage reduces the viral load for infectivity (Peterson and Rao 1989).

Chapter 5: Damaged Goods

1. "The immune system of most healthy people is able to suppress HPV within a few months" however, "HPV can have a long latency period in the body, where no symptoms appear for months or even years after infection" (ASHA Server 2006c).

Chapter 6: Sexual Healing

1. "A Pap smear is a microscopic examination of cells scraped from the uterine cervix;" in contrast, "during colposcopy, a magnifying instrument is used to view the vagina and uterine cervix," which allows for inspection of a greater area and facilitates biopsies of cervical and vaginal tissue (JAMA Server 2001).

2. The optimal mode of treatment "is local destruction of HPV-related lesions:" Cells infected with HPV DNA that are left at the treatment site will likely promote recurrence (Keller et al.1995, 357–358).

3. Almost all of the women with herpes mentioned the pain of urinating during an outbreak. Rebecca discovered on her own she could use a small spray bottle of water to spray on the area as she was urinating to dilute the acidity and lessen the pain of her sores.

Chapter 7: Reintegrating the Sexual Self

1. This polyurethane sheath, closed at one end and held open at the other with a plastic ring at the edge of the opening, is inserted in the vagina, with

the ring and the last inch of the sheath remaining outside to better protect against skin-to-skin contact.

2. While viruses such as herpes and hepatitis can survive briefly on surfaces such as toilet seats, an individual would have to make contact with the virus with their genital skin or other vulnerable tissue (such as abraded skin on thighs) to contract the virus from a toilet seat.

3. "If a pregnant woman has active herpes during delivery, her child may become infected, leading to retardation or death; this possibility, however, can be avoided by caesarean section" (Brandt 1987, 180).

4. Ingrid created "Matt" as a pseudonym for this person.

Chapter 8: From Personal Tragedies to Social Change

1. The Centers for Disease Control and Prevention's Advisory Committee on Immunization Practices (ACIP) recommended "universal administration" in 11 to 12 year-old girls and also allowed medical practitioners to immunize girls as young as nine and women as old as 26 years of age (CDC ACIP 2007).

2. March 2007 issue of *The American Journal of Obstetrics and Gynecology*

3. Accessed online http://intl-caonline.amcancersoc.org/cgi/content/full/57/1/7 (May 30, 2007); *CA: A Cancer Journal for Clinicians* 2007, 57:7–28.

4. Future research should focus on men living with chronic STDs and compare the gendered dimensions of this type of illness experience.

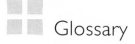

Glossary

abortion: The spontaneous or induced expulsion of the product of conception between fertilization and birth.

abstinence: The act or practice of refraining from sexual activity.

adolescence: The period of psychological and social development between the beginning of puberty and adulthood.

AIDS: A set of maladies resulting from the immune system damage caused by the human immunodeficiency virus (HIV).

anogenital warts: Usually flesh-colored growths on the genital skin and linings of the vagina, cervix, rectum, and urethra; most often caused by types of human papillomavirus (HPV) that are different from the types that can cause cervical cancer.

ascribed traits: Innate characteristics over which an individual has limited to no control, such as ethnicity or gender.

asymptomatic carrier: A person infected with, or a carrier of, a disease that nonetheless shows no symptoms.

attitude: The tendency to behave or think in a certain way.

auto-ethnography: A social research method where the researcher documents and analyzes their own life-experiences.

auxiliary traits: Term created by sociologist Everett Hughes to describe the set of traits that accompany one's master status; see *master status*.

avoidance: Mentally or physically withdrawing from situations that cause distress.

behavior: The actions of a person.

bias: A prejudice or predisposition that prevents objective assessment.

bisexuality: Being emotionally and sexually attracted to both males and females.

casual sex: Sex with someone not well know outside of a relationship.

cathartic disclosure: A personal revelation that produces therapeutic effects.

celibacy: The practice of refraining from engaging in sexual activity.

cervical cancer: Invasive cancer of the lower part of the uterus.

cervical dysplasia or cervical intraepithelial neoplasia (CIN): The presence of abnormal cells in the lining of the cervix that have changed in appearance; the more severe the abnormality, the more likely the possibility of developing cervical cancer.

cervix: The lower, narrow end of the uterus that joins it to the top of the vaginal canal.

cervical cancer: Cancer of the cervix, most often caused by the cervical cells becoming infected by certain types of human papillomavirus (HPV), which can cause abnormal cells to develop in the lining of the cervix. If not detected early and removed by treatment(s), then these abnormal cells can become precancerouss and ultimately cancer.

cervical lesions: Usually flat growths of abnormal cells on the lining of the cervix; typically caused by the HPV infection.

Cesarean section (C-section): A method of delivering a baby that occurs through an incision in the mother's abdominal and uterine walls.

Chlamydia: A sexually transmitted disease caused by the *Chlamydia trachmatis* bacterium; also known as Chlamydial infection.

chronic STD: An incurable sexually transmitted disease.

clitoris: The female arousal center located externally above the opening of the vagina.

colposcopy: Examination of the cells lining the vaginal canal and cervix by means of a specially designed microscope, known as a colposcope.

communication: The process of exchanging information such as words, gestures, and movements to establish human contact, or attempt to affect attitudes and behaviors.

complete member: A social researcher engaged in participant observation research who is regarded as a full part of the community they are studying.

compliance: The act of following the instructions of health care providers.

condom (male condom): A sheath of latex, polyurethane, or processed animal tissue that is placed over an erect penis to prevent semen transmission.

conflict: A disagreement or inconsistency in goals within or between people.

construct validity: The extent to which a measure or category accurately assesses the underlying theoretical construct it is supposed to measure.

contraception: A device used to prevent conception.

covering: Concealing one's deviant status by means of deception in order to avoid deviant stigma.

cryosurgery: Medical application of liquid nitrogen to freeze and, thereby, kill abnormal cells.

date rape: The act of coercing a dating partner into sexual activity without that partner's consent.

demographics: The characteristics of human populations aggregated through statistics.

deviance: Behavior, attitudes, or conditions counter to the norms of a given culture, which results in negative social sanctions.

deviant: A person who has been interactionally labeled as practicing a form of deviance. See *deviance*.

disclosing: Telling others about one's deviance or making it more visible.

disease: An impairment of bodily function.

disidentifiers: Objects and actions employed to mask one's association with a deviant group, thereby avoiding deviant stigma.

dynamics of exclusion: A term first used by sociologist Charles Lemert to describe the process of being ostracized from a social group; this process commonly occurs when one has been labeled as deviant.

dysplasia: See *cervical dysplasia*.

efficacy: The ability to produce a desired result or effect.

epidemic: The emergence of a new disease or a sudden rise in the rate of a known disease.

epidemiology: The branch of medicine that studies the causes and mitigation of disease.

erection: The rigidifying of an organ, like the penis or clitoris, through vascongestion.

ethnicity: Traits, experiences, and affinity with a particular national, cultural, or racial group.

female condom: A polyurethane sheath, open at one end with a flexible ring in the closed end, that covers the cervix, walls of the vaginal canal, and part of the vulva; used to prevent conception and sexually transmitted diseases.

fetus: Medical term for an unborn vertebrate from eight weeks after conception to birth.

gender: The condition and performance of being regarded as female or male.

gender identity: The self-classification into a gender category.

gender role: The set of traits and roles each society identifies with men and women.

genital herpes: An STD that results from contracting the the herpes simplex virus (HSV), usually Type 2 (HSV).

genital warts: See *anogenital warts.*

genitals: The external male and female reproductive and sexual organs.

gonorrhea: A sexually transmitted disease produced by contracting the *Neisseria gonorrhoeae* bacterium.

grounded theory: A methodology where researchers develop theories about social phenomena from analysis of empirical data.

heterosexuality: Sexual and emotional attraction to persons of the other sex.

HIV (human immunodeficiency virus): A retrovirus that infects T-cells of the human immune system and thereby causes HIV disease.

HIV disease: A disease in humans resulting from HIV infection that gradually damages a body's immune system and most often leads to death years after the initial infection.

HIV-seropositive: A classification that indicates a person's blood contains antibodies to HIV infections.

homophobia: An irrational fear or revulsion towards gay and lesbian people.

homosexuality: Attraction to persons of the same sex.

HPV (human papillomavirus): Any of the strains of *Human papillomavirus* that cause anogenital warts, cervical lesions, and/or abnormal cellular changes; it has been casually linked to cancer of the cervix, vagina, vulva, penis, anus, and certain oral, head, and neck cancers.

HSV (herpes simplex virus): See *genital herpes.*

hysterectomy: The surgical removal of part or all of the uterus.

identity dilemma: A crisis in self-concept resulting from loss of valued attributes, physical functions, social roles, and/or personal pursuits; often occurs as a result of serious illness.

identity transformation: A reframing of how an individual views him/herself.

illness: The state of being in an unhealthy condition and the social experience therein.

illness behavior: An ill person's responses to symptoms, such as seeking medical assistance.

immoral patient: Third stage in the sexual-self transformation process of women with chronic STDs; involves experiencing a medical practitioner's delivery of an STD diagnoses as conveying health, moral, and social stigma.

impotency: A persistent inability in a male to maintain or attain an erection.

informed consent: The practice of making the decision to participate in medical research, or to receive medical treatment, with full understanding of the potential risks and benefits.

incest: Sexual intercourse between close relatives.

infertility: The inability to produce offspring.

intrapersonal: Occurring within the individual self.

interactionist: An adherent of symbolic interactionism theory, which emphasizes the ways in which people give meaning to their social worlds.

interpersonal: Relating to interactions between two or more people.

introspection: Self-examination of one's observation or examination of one's own thoughts and feelings.

labia majora: The two outer folds of skin that lie on either side of the vaginal opening and form the clitoral hood.

labia minora: The two inner folds of the skin within the entrance of the vagina and enclosed within the labia majora.

Loop electrocautery excision procedures (LEEP): A procedure used for the treatment of cervical intraepithelial neoplasia (CIN) that uses an electrified wire loop to remove abnormal tissue.

master status: Term created by sociologist Everett Hughes to denote an individual's dominant identity, which affects the ways in which others relate to that person.

masturbation: The manipulation of the genitals by oneself for one's own sexual pleasure.

menstrual cycle: The recurring process of physiological changes, during which the uterus is readied for implantation of a fertilized ovum.

minority group: Any group differing from the majority of a population that is considered inferior and has little power relative to the majority group.

molestation: Unwelcome, unwarranted, and improper sexual acts.

moral status: Society's moral evaluation of an individual, based on their perceived membership with a social group.

mortality: Death.

normalize: To make something appear consistent with a standard or norm.

norms: Behavior regarded as typical and appropriate in a given society.

opinion: A individual view one believes to be true.

oral sex: Sexual contact of a partner's genitals or anus with the mouth and/or tongue.

orgasm: The pleasurable sensation experienced at the peak of sexual excitement, usually resulting from stimulation of the sex organs and usually including ejaculation in males.

os: The cervical opening.

other-directed: Person guided by external influences rather than one's own needs and preferences.

outpatient: Patient receiving medical treatment and or undergoing medical procedures when not formally hospitalized or kept for overnight observation.

Pap test/smear: Method of testing for cervical cancer by scraping cell samples from the lining of the cervix and examining them under a microscope.

pandemic: A worldwide epidemic. See *epidemic*.

passing: The act of concealing deviance in order to fit in with non-deviant people and avoid the deviant stigma.

penis: The external male organ used for urination and sex.

perineum: In male and female human beings, an area of soft tissue in front of the anus that covers the muscles and ligaments of the pelvic floor.

preventive disclosure: Revealing one's deviant status to persons considered normal of a deviant attribute in order to prevent harm to self or others.

prejudice: A bias towards or against individuals, based on their membership in a particular group.

prevalence: The number of incidences of a particular pathology within a population at a particular point in time.

primary deviance: Sociologist Edwin Lemert created this term to refer to the first type of deviance, in which an individual engages, but does not result in that person being publicly caught or labeled as a deviant.

profession: The body of persons engaged in an occupation or calling that requires specialized knowledge or training.

prostitution: The exchange of sexual behavior/contact for money, services, and/or goods.

puberty: The stage of human development when an individual becomes capable of sexual reproduction.

pubic lice: Parasitic insects found in the genital area of humans that can be spread during sexual intercourse; sometimes referred to by slang term "crabs."

punch biopsies: A diagnostic test on abnormal skin growths that removes a small disk-shaped piece of skin tissue using a sharp, hollow device.

qualitative research methods: Forms of collecting and analyzing data, which emphasize the meanings of persona experiences, perceptions, and social actions.

random sample: A subset of a larger group selected by or chosen in an unbiased way and expected to represent a population.

rape: An act of sexual intercourse against a person's will and involving coercion.

rates: The degree or comparative extent of a phenomenon in a given population.

reintegrating the sexual self: Sixth stage in the sexual-self transformation process of women with chronic STDs; involves reconciling an illness experience, within an individual's sexual self concept, and the necessary transformations of one's sexual self.

representativeness: The practice of selecting subjects for study that accurately exemplifys a population of interest.

respiratory papillomatosis: HPV-caused lesions in the larynx and trachea, found in a small number of babies born to mothers with HPV.

scissors excision: A procedure to remove genital warts by use of a pair of fine scissors.

secondary deviance: Sociologist Edwin Lemert created this term to refer to the second stage, in what sociologist Howard Becker has termed a "deviant career:" When an individual has been caught and publicly labeled as a deviant. This results in others interacting with that person as a deviant and, ultimately, in the individual seeing his/herself as deviant.

secret self: Term coined by social theorist James Dowd coined this term to designate a realm of behavior that one engages in away from the public; a private self.

self-disclosure: The conscious and unconscious revelation of personal information that might be concealed because of fear of being judged by others.

semen: A yellow-white fluid containing sperm, ejaculated from the penis, during orgasm or nocturnal emission.

sex: Term used to describe two groups, categorized as male and female, and to the chromosomal structure, genitalia, hormones etc. that distinguish males from females.

sexism: Preconceived assumptions about people based on their sex, typically favoring men over women.

sexual assault: Physical sexual contact without voluntary consent.

sexual harassment: Unwelcome sexual attention that creates a hostile organizational environment for the victim.

sexual healing: The fifth stage in the sexual-self transformation process of women with chronic STDs; involves experiencing the interpersonal, physical, emotional, and financial challenges of treatment.

sexual health: The condition of physical and mental well-being as it pertains to sexuality.

sexual intercourse: The human form of copulation, including any form of sexual behavior that involves insertion/penetration.

sexual interest: Being attracted to others for sexual or erotic purposes.

sexual invincibility: First stage in the sexual-self transformation process of women with chronic STDs; involves believing that one's sexual health is not vulnerable to disease.

sexual orientation: One's predisposition towards the attractiveness, or lack thereof, of sex partners; usually categorized as asexual, homosexual, heterosexual, or bisexual.

sexual self: An aspect of identity that is typically private and is formed by emotions, cognitions, evaluations, and memories of sexual experiences.

sexually transmitted diseases (STDs): Infections caused by diseases, which have a significant possibility of being transmitted through person-to-person sexual contact.

sexually transmitted infections (STIs): See *sexually transmitted diseases (STDs).*

sexuality: Elements in human beings that relate to sexual attraction and expression.

snowball sampling: A technique for constructing a research sample, whereby individuals are included based on their acquaintance with members of the original sample.

social class: Hierarchical classifications within a society, or culture of individuals, or groups based on characteristics, such as race, religion, education, income and/or occupational status.

social construction: A phenomena in a society or culture that exists because members of the social group agree to behave as if it is true, as opposed to something that is objectively true.

social control: Means used by a social group to regulate individual and group behavior, such that individuals conform to the norms of that group.

social control agents: Individuals, groups, or institutions with the authority to enforce social norms.

social influence model: A theory of behavior that suggests peer norms play a significant role in structuring human action.

social mores: Norms or customs within a society that derive from established practices and traditions and are thus strongly held.

social psychology: Within the disciplines of either psychology or sociology, the study of the behavior of individuals and groups engaged in face-to-face social interaction.

sociocultural: That which refers to the combination of social and cultural elements.

socioeconomic: That which refers to the combination of social and economic elements, such as classifying individuals on both their income and occupational status.

spoiled identity: A term developed by sociologist Erving Goffman to describe a sense of social self that individuals develop when they experience a reduced sense of control as a result of being labeled a "deviant" and obtaining a damaged reputation.

STD anxiety: The second stage in the sexual-self transformation process of women with chronic STDs; involves women's experiences of initial symptoms, or practitioners' suggestions of possible infection, which leads to replacing their prior feelings of *sexual invincibility* with suspicion and fear.

stereotypes: An over-simplistic, yet conventional, set of assumptions about members of a particular group.

stigma: An individual attribute that, if known, would place an individual at risk of being labeled as deviant.

stigma symbols: Behaviors or objects that would link someone to their deviant status.

stigma transference: A term coined by sociologist Adina Nack to describe the unconscious process in which the individual transfers stigma to real or imaginary others in a failed effort to reduce their anxiety.

stigmata: The plural form of stigma.

stress: Outcome of one being in situations, whereby the individual experiences a condition of extreme difficulty, pressure, or strain and responds both psychologically and physiologically.

structure: The numerous parts of society that are held or put together in a particular way and affect individual choices.

survey research: A research method where information is gathered from a smaller sub-group to make inferences about the group as a whole.

symbolic interactionism: A theoretical perspective that suggests people's behavior is structured by the meanings they develop toward specific acts. These meanings are derived from social interaction and interpretation.

syphilis: An STD resulting from contracting the *Treponema pallidum* bacterium.

tertiary deviance: Sociologist John Kitsuse added this stage onto Lemert's first two to delineate a final stage that not all deviants reach: When an individual not only accepts their deviant status, but also embraces their deviant status, by rejecting others' definition of it as deviant.

theory construction: The practice of developing a set of principles for explaining a group of facts or phenomena, with the aim of enhancing its understanding, or making predictions about future behavior.

total pattern: A sequence of events that holds true for a group studied.

turning-point moment: Sociologist Anselm Strauss created this term to describe an event that makes one challenge previously held assumptions.

uterus: A hollow, pear-shaped, muscular organ of the female reproductive system in which the fetus develops during pregnancy.

vagina: A flexible, muscular organ that leads from the opening of the vulva to the cervix that serves as the passage through which an infant is born.

venereal disease: A historical term for any of several diseases transmitted through sexual intercourse; see *sexually transmitted diseases (STDs)*.

vulva: The external female genital organs, including the vaginal opening, clitoris, and labia.

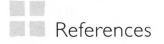

References

Adler, Patricia A. and Peter Adler. 1987. *Membership Roles in Field Research.* Newbury Park,CA: Sage.

Adler, Patricia A. and Peter Adler. 2006. *Constructions of Deviance: Social Power, Context, and Interaction (Fifth Edition).* Belmont, CA: Thomson Wadsworth.

American Social Health Association Server. 2006a. "Quick Facts about HPV." *National HPV and Cervical Cancer Resource Center:* www.ashastd.org/hpv/hpvrc/fact1.html

American Social Health Association Server. 2006b. "Quick Facts about Herpes." *National Herpes Resource Center:* www.ashastd.org/herpes/hrc/info1.html

American Social Health Association Server. 2006c. "Fact Sheet on HPV." *National HPV Cervical Cancer Resource Center:* http://www.ashastd.org/pdfs/HPV_factsheet.pdf

Bassett Mary. T. and M. Mhloyi. 1991. "Women and AIDS in Zimbabwe: the making of an epidemic. *International Journal of Health Services,* 21, 1:143–56.

Beadnell, Blair, Baker, Sharon A., Morrison, Diane M., Huang, Bu, Stielstra, Sorrel, and Susan Stoner. 2006. "Change Trajectories in Women's STD/HIV Risk Behaviors Following Intervention." *Preventive Science,* 7:321–331.

Best, Joel and David F. Luckenbill. 1980. "The Social Organization of Deviants." *Social Problems,* 28,1:14–31.

Best, Joel. 2006. "Deviance: The Constructionist Stance." In Patricia A. Adler and Peter Adler (eds.) Constructions of Deviance: Social Power, Context, and Interactions, pp. 92–95. Belmont, CA: Thomson/Wadsworth.

Bettoli, E.J. 1982. "Herpes: facts and fallacies." American Journal of Nursing: 924–29.

Biernacki, Patrick, and Dan Waldorf. 1981. "Snowball Sampling." Sociological Research Methods, 10:141–63.

Blumer, Herbert. 1969. Symbolic interactionism: perspective and method. Berkeley: University of California Press.

———. 1973. "A Note on Symbolic Interactionism." American Sociological Review, 38, 6:797–98.

Bourdieu, Pierre. 1986. On symbols and society. Chicago: University of Chicago Press.

Brandt, Allan M. 1987. No magic bullet: a social history of venereal disease in the United States since 1880. New York: Oxford University Press.

———. 1997. "Behavior, Disease, and Health in the Twentieth Century United States: The Moral Valence of Individual Risk." In A. Brandt and Paul Rozin (eds.) Morality and Health, pp. New York: Routledge.

Braun V., and N. Gavey. 1999. "'With the best of reasons': Cervical cancer prevention policy and the suppression of sexual risk factor information. Social Science & Medicine, 38: 1463–74.

Breakwell, Glynis M. and Lynne J. Millward. 1997. "Sexual self-concept and sexual risk-taking." Journal of Adolescence, 20:29–41.

Breitkopf, Carmen Radecki. 2004. "The Theoretical Basis of Stigma as Applied to Genital Herpes." HERPES, 11, 1:4–7.

Brody, Jane E. May 15, 2007. "HPV Vaccine: Few Risks, Many Benefits." The New York Times. Retrieved, May 21, 2007, from http://www.nytimes.com

Buller, M.K. and D.B. Buller. 1987. "Physician's Communication Style and Patient Satisfaction." Journal of Health and Social Behavior, 13:347–59.

Centers for Disease Control and Prevention (CDC), Division of Sexually Transmitted Disease Prevention. 1999. Prevention of Genital HPV Infection and Sequelae: Report of an External Consultants Meeting. Atlanta, GA: U.S. Department of Health and Human Services.

———. 2000. "Common STDs." National Center for HIV, STD & TB Prevention: www.cdcnpin.org/std/common.htm.

———. 2002. HPV communication and outreach (Report No. 2001-Q-00133 [E-40]). Atlanta, GA: ORC Macro International.

———. 2006. "HPV Vaccine: Questions and Answers." August 2006: accessed online May 31, 2007. http://www.cdc.gov/std/hpv/STDFact-HPV-vaccine.htm

———. 2007. "Recommended Immunization Schedules for Persons Aged 0–18 Years—United States, 2007." MMWR Weekly. January 5, 2007 / 55(51):Q1-Q4.

Charmaz, Kathy. 1994. "Identity Dilemmas in Chronically Ill Men." *Sociological Quarterly*, 35:269–88.

———. 1995. "Learning Grounded Theory." In Jonathon Smith, Rom Harré, and Luk Van Langenhove (eds.) *Rethinking Methods in Psychology*, pp. 27–49. London: Sage Publications.

———. 2000. "Experiencing Chronic Illness." In Albrecht, Fitzpatrick, and Scrimshaw (eds.) *Handbook of Social Studies in Health and Medicine*, pp. 277–92. London: Sage Publications.

Charmaz, Kathy, and Virginia Olesen. 1997. "Ethnographic research in medical sociology: Its foci and distinctive contributions." *Sociological Methods and Research*, 25:452–94.

Cline, J. Steven. 2006. "Sexually Transmitted Diseases: Will this Problem Ever Go Away?" *North Carolina Medical Journal*. 67, 5: 353–58.

Conrad, Peter, and Joseph W. Schneider. 1980. *Deviance and Medicalization: From Badness to Sickness*. St. Louis, MO: The C.V. Mosby Company.

Cooley, Charles H. [1902] 1964. *Human nature and the social order*. New York: Schocken Books.

Cranson, Denis A. and Sandra L. Caron. 1998. "An Investigation of the Effects of HIV on the Sex Lives of Infected Individuals." *AIDS Education and Prevention*, 10, 6:506–22.

Crites, Stephen L. 1986. "Storytime: Recollecting the past and projecting the future." In T.R. Sarbin (ed.) *Narrative psychology: The storied nature of human conduct*, pp. 152–73. New York: Praeger.

Daly, Mary B. and Barabara S. Hulka. 1975. "Talking with the Doctor, 2" *Journal of Communication*, 25:148–52.

Davenport-Hines, R. 1991. *Sex, Death and Punishment: Attitudes to Sex and Sexuality in Britain since the Renaissance*. London: W. Heinemann/Reed Books.

Davidson, Roger. 1994. "Venereal Disease, Sexual Morality, and Public Health in Interwar Scotland." *Journal of the History of Sexuality*, 5, 2:267–94.

Delaney, Janice, Mary Jane Lupton, and Emily Toth. 1988. *The Curse: a Cultural History of Menstruation*. Urbana: University of Illinois Press.

Dempsey, Amanda F., Zimet, G.D., Davis, R.L. and L. Koutsky. 2006. "Factors that are Associated with Parental Acceptance of Human Papillomavirus Vaccines: A Randomized Intervention Study of Written Information About HPV." *Pediatrics*, 117, 5:1486–1493.

Dihn, Tri A. and Michelle F. Benoit. 2007. "Human Papillomavirus Vaccine: Progress and the Future." *Expert Opinion on Biological Therapy*, 7, 4:479–485.

Dock, Lavinia. 1910. *Hygiene and Morality: A Manual for Nurses and Others, Giving an Outline of the Medical, Social and Legal Aspects of the Venereal Diseases*. New York: G.P. Putnam's Sons.

Dowd, James J. 1996. "An Act Made Perfect in Habit: The Self in the Postmodern Age." *Current Perspectives in Social Theory*, 16:237–63.

Ehrenreich, Barbara and Deirdre English. 1973. *Complaints and Disorders: The sexual politics of sickness.* Old Westbury, NY: Feminist Press.

Ellis, Carolyn. 1991. "Sociological Introspection and Emotional Experience." *Symbolic Interaction,* 14, 1:23–50.

Eng, Thomas and William Butler. 1997. *The Hidden Epidemic: Confronting Sexually Transmitted Diseases.* Washington, DC: National Academy Press.

Eyre, S. L., Davis, E. W., & Peacock, B. 2001. Moral Argumentation in Adolescents' Commentaries About Sex." *Culture, Health, and Sexuality, 3,* 1: 1–17.

Family Research Council (FRC). 2007a. "Clarification of 2005 Family Research Council Media Remarks on HPV Vaccine." Feb. 12, 2007 (Accessed online May 31, 2007) http://www.frc.org/get.cfm?i=LH07B02&f=WX06K03

Family Research Council (FRC). 2007b. "States Taking Their Best Shot at HPV." April 23, 2007 (Accessed online May 31, 2007) http://www.frc.org/get.cfm?i=WA07D37#WA07D37

Fernando, M. Daniel. 1993. *AIDS and Intravenous Drug Use: the Influence of Morality, Politics, Social Science, and Race in the Making of a Tragedy.* London: Praeger.

Fisher, J.D. 1988. "Possible effects of reference group-based social influence on AIDS risk behavior and AIDS prevention. *American Psychologist,* 43:914–20.

Ford, Carol A. and Anna-Barbara Moscicki. 1995. "Control of Sexually Transmitted Diseases in Adolescents: The Clinician's Role." *Advances in Pediatric Infectious Diseases,* 10:263–305.

Foucault, Michel. 1978. *The History of Sexuality, volume 1.* New York: Pantheon.

Frank, Arthur W. 1991. *At the Will of the Body.* Boston, MA: Houghton Mifflin Company.

———. 1993. "The Rhetoric of Self-change: Illness Experience as Narrative." *The Sociological Quarterly* 34, 1: 39–52.

———. 1997. "Ethics and the Postmodern Crisis of Medicine." In Paul A. Komesaroff (ed.) *Expanding the Horizons of Bioethics,* pp. 27–9. Melbourne, Australia: Australia Bioethics Association.

———. 1998. "Just Listening: Narrative and Deep Illness." *Families, Systems & Health,*16, 3:197–216.

Friedman, Allison L. and Hilda Shepeard. 2007. "Exploring the Knowledge, Attitudes, Beliefs, and Communication Preferences of the General Public Regarding HPV: Findings From the CC Focus Group Research and Implications for Practice." *Health Education & Behavior* 34(3):471–485.

Garfinkel, Harold. 1956. "Conditions of Successful Degradation Ceremonies." *American Journal of Sociology,* 61:420–24.

Gaussot, Ludovic. 1998. Representations of Alcoholism & the Social Construction of "Good Drinking," *Sciences Sociales et Sante*, 16, 1:5–42.

Gilman, Sander L. 1988. *Disease and Representation: Images of Illness from Madness to AIDS*. Ithaca, NY: Cornell University Press.

Glaser, Barney G. 1978. *Theoretical sensitivity*. Mill Valley, CA: Sociological Press.

Glaser, Barney G., and Anselm L. Strauss. 1967. *The Discovery of Grounded Theory: Strategies for Qualitative Research*. Chicago: Aldine.

Goffman, Erving. 1959. "The Moral Career of the Mental Patient." *Psychiatry*, 22,2: 123–42.

————. 1963. *Stigma: Notes on the Management of Spoiled Identity*. Englewood Cliffs, NJ: Prentice Hall.

————. 1972. *Strategic Interaction*. New York: Ballantine.

Griffith R.S., Walsh, D.E., Myrmel, K.H., Thompson, R.W. and A. Behforooz. 1987. "Success of L-lysine Therapy in Frequently Recurrent Herpes Simplex Infection. Treatment and Prophylaxis." *Dermatologica*, 175, 4:183–90.

Grove, Kathleen A., Donald P. Kelly, and Judith Liu. 1997. "But Nice Girls Don't Get It: Women, Symbolic Capital, and the Social Construction of AIDS." *Journal of Contemporary Ethnography*, 26, 3: 317–37.

Harding, Sandra, ed. 1987. *Feminism and Methodology*. Bloomington: Indiana University Press.

Hayano, D.M. 1979. "Auto-ethnography: paradigms, problem, and prospects." *Human Organization*, 38:99–104.

Herman, Nancy J. 1993. "Return to Sender: Reintegrative Stigma-Management Strategies of Ex-Psychiatric Patients." *Journal of Contemporary Ethnography*, 22, 3:295–330.

Hermans, Hubert J.M. 1996. "Voicing the Self: From Information Processing to Dialogical Interchange." *Psychological Bulletin*, 119, 1:31–50.

Honey, Karen. 2006. "HPV Vaccine Gets a Shot in the Arm." *The Journal of Clinical Intervention*. 116, 12: 3087.

Hughes, Everett. 1945. "Dilemmas and Contradictions of Status." *American Journal of Sociology*, March:353–59.

James, William. [1890] 1902. *The principles of psychology* (Vol. 1). London: Macmillan.

Joanisse, Leanne. 1999. "Fat Bias in the Delivery of Health Care." *Annual Meeting of the American Sociological Association*: Chicago, IL.

Journal of the American Medical Association. 2001. "Human Papillomavirus and Genital Warts." *JAMA Women's Health: Sexually Transmitted Disease Information Center*: www.ama-assn.org/special/std/support/educate/stdhpv.htm

Karp, David A. 1992. "Illness Ambiguity and the Search for Meaning: A Case Study of a Self-Help Group for Affective Disorders." *Journal of Contemporary Ethnography*, 21, 2:139–70.

Keller, Mary L., Mims, L. Fern, and Judith J. Egan. 1992. "Disease-related stressors and need of persons newly diagnosed with human papillomavirus. Paper presented at the 16th *Annual Research Conference of the Midwest Nursing Research Society*, Chicago.

———. 1995. "Genital Human Papillomavirus Infection: Common but Not Trivial." *Health Care for Women International*, 16:351–64.

Keller, Mary L., von Sadovszky, V., Pankratz, B., and J. Hermsen. 2000. "Self-disclosure of HPV infection to sexual partners." *Western Journal of Nursing Research*, 22:285–96.

Kelly, Michael. 1992 "Self, identity and radical surgery." *Sociology of Health & Illness*, 14, 3:390–415.

Kitsuse, John. 1962 "Societal Reactions to Deviant Behavior: Problems of Theory and Method." *Social Problems*, 9:247–56.

———. 1980. "Coming Out All Over: Deviants and the Politics of Social Problems."*Social Problems* 28:1–13.

Kelly, Michael. 1992. "Self, identity and radical surgery." *Sociology of Health & Illness*, 14, 3:390–415.

Kimberlin, David W. "Neonatal Herpes Simplex Infection." 2004. *Clinical Microbiology Reviews*, 17, 1: 1–13.

Korsch, Barbara M., Ethel K. Gozzi, and Vida F. Francis. 1968. Gaps in Doctor-Patient Communication, *Pediatrics,* 42:855–70.

Korsch, Barbara M. and Vida F. Negrete. 1972. "Doctor-Patient Communication." *Scientific American*, 227:66–74.

Lavin, Bebe, Marie Haug, Linda Liska Belgrave, and Naomi Breslau. 1987. "Change in Student Physicians' Views on Authority Relationships with Patients." *Journal of Health and Social Behavior,* 28, 3:258–72.

Lawless, Sonia, Susan Kippax, and June Crawford. 1996. "Dirty, Diseased and Undeserving: the Positioning of HIV Positive Women." *Social Science and Medicine,* 43,9:1371–77.

Lemert, Edwin. 1951. *Social Pathology.* New York: McGraw-Hill.

———. 1962. "Paranoia and the dynamics of exclusion." *Sociometry,* 25:2–20.

———. 1967. *Human Deviance, Social Problems and Social Control.* Englewood Cliffs, NJ: Prentice-Hall.

Leonardo, Cecelia and Joan C. Chrisler. 1992. "Women and Sexually Transmitted Diseases." *Women & Health,* 18, 4:1–15.

Lichtenstein, Bronwen. 2003. "Stigma as a barrier to treatment of sexually transmitted infection in the American deep south: issues of race, gender and poverty." *Social Science & Medicine,* 57:2435–2445.

Lock, Margaret and P. Kaufert. 1998. *Pragmatic Women and Body Politics.* Cambridge: Cambridge University Press.

Lock, Margaret. 2000. "Accounting for Disease and Distress: Morals of the Normal and Abnormal." In Albrecht, Fitzpatrick, and Scrimshaw (eds.)

Handbook of Social Studies in Health and Medicine, pp. 259–76. London: Sage Publications.

Lorber, Judith. 1993. "Believing is Seeing: Biology as Ideology." *Gender and Society,* 7, 4:568–81.

Lowery, Shearon A. and Charles V. Wetli. 1982. "Sexual Asphyxia: A Neglected Area of Study." *Deviant Behavior,* 3, 1:19–39.

Luker, Kristin. 1998. "Sex, Social Hygiene, and the State: The Double-Edged Sword of Social Reform." *Theory and Society,* 27, 5:601–34.

Mahood, Linda. 1990. "The Magdalene's Friend: Prostitution and Social Control in Glasgow,1869–90." *Women's Studies International Forum,* 13, 1/2:49–61.

Mancuso, James C., and Theodore R. Sarbin. 1983. "The self-narrative in the enactment of roles." In T.R. Sarbin and K. Scheibe (eds.) *Studies in social identity,* pp. 254–73. NewYork: Praeger.

Manzo, John F. 2004. "On the Sociology and Social Organization of Stigma: Some Ethnomethodological Insights." *Human Studies,* 27:401–16.

Marshall, Gordon. 1994. *The Concise Oxford Dictionary of Sociology.* Oxford: Oxford University Press.

Matthews, Eric. 1988. "AIDS and Sexual Morality." *Bioethics,* 2, 2:118–28.

McAdams, Dan P. 1996. *The stories we live by: personal myths and the making of the self.* New York: Guilford Press.

Mead, George Herbert. 1934. *Mind, self, and society.* Chicago: University of Chicago Press.

Mechanic, David (ed.). 1982. *Symptoms, Illness Behavior, and Help-Seeking.* New York: Prodist.

———. 1989. *Painful Choices: Research and Essays on Health Care.* New Brunswick, NJ: Transaction Publishers.

Melville, J., Sniffen, S., Crosby, R., Salazar, L., Whittington, W., Dithmer-Schreck, D., DiClemente, R., and A. Wald. 2003. "Psychosocial impact of serological diagnosis of herpes simplex virus type 2: a qualitative assessment." *Sexually Transmitted Infections,* 79:280–85.

Meyer-Weitz, A., Reddy, P., Weijts, W., van den Borne, B., and G. Kok. 1998. "The socio-cultural contexts of sexually transmitted diseases in South Africa: implications for healtheducation programmes." *AIDS Care,* 10, 1:539–55.

Mort, F. 1987. *Dangerous Sexualities: Medico-Moral Politics in England since 1830.* London: Routledge & Kegan Paul.

Nechas, Eileen and Denise Foley. 1994. *Unequal Treatment: What You Don't Know About HowWomen Are Mistreated by the Medical Community.* New York: Simon & Schuster.

Oakley, Ann. 1981. "Interviewing Women: A Contradiction in Terms" In Helen Roberts, ed. *Doing Feminist Research,* pp. 30–63. London: Routledge, Kegan and Paul.

O'Byrne, Patrick and Dave Holmes. 2005. "Re-Evaluating Current Public Health Policy: Alternative Public Health Nursing Approaches to Sexually Transmitted Infection Testing for Teens and Males who Have Sex with Males." *Public Health Nursing* 22, 6:523–28.

Parry, J. 2007. Vaccinating against cervical cancer. *Bulletin of the World Health Organization*, 85, 89–90.

Partridge, J.M., & Koutsky, L.A. 2006. "Genital human papillomavirus infection in men." *The Lancet Infectious Diseases*, 6, 1:21–31.

Peterson, I. M. and R. Rao. 1989. "Genital warts: Newly discovered consequences of an ancient disease." *Postgraduate Medicine*, 86:197–204.

Pitts, Marian, Margaret Bowman and John McMaster. 1995. "Reactions to Repeated STD Infections: Psychosocial Aspects and Gender Issues in Zimbabwe." *Social Science and Medicine*, 40, 9:1299–1304.

Plummer, Ken. 1995. *Telling Sexual Stories: Power, change, and social worlds.* London: Routledge.

Plumridge, E.W., and S.J. Chetwynd. 1998. "The Moral Universe of Injecting Drug Users in the Era of AIDS: Sharing Injecting Equipment and the Protection of Moral Standing." *AIDS Care*, 10, 6:723–33.

Pyrce, Anthony. 1998. "Theorizing the Pox: A Missing Sociology of VD." Presented to the *International Sociological Association*.

Radley, Alan. 1994. *Making Sense of Illness: The Social Psychology of Health and Disease.* London: Sage Publications.

Raine, T.R., Harper, C.C., C.H. Rocca, Fischer, R. and N. Padian. 2005. "Direct Access to Emergency Contraception Through Pharmacies and Effect on Unintended Pregnancy and STIs: A Randomized Controlled Trial." *JAMA* 293: 54–62.

Ray, Laurence J. 1989. "AIDS as a Moral Metaphor. An Analysis of the Politics of the Third Epidemic." *Archives Europeennes de Sociologie*, 30, 2:243–73.

Reinharz, Shulamit. 1990. *Feminist Methods in Social Research.* Oxford: Oxford University Press.

Roth, Julius A. 1972. "Some Contingencies of the Moral Evaluation and Control of Clientele: The Case of Hospital Emergency Staff." *American Journal of Sociology*, 77, 5:839–56.

Reiser, Christa. 1986. "Herpes: A Physical and Moral Dilemma." *College Student Journal*, 20, 3:260–269.

Rogers, Susan Matthews. 1999. "Sexual Behavior and Risk of Sexually Transmitted Diseases: Do Community CharacteriSTDcs Moderate the Relationship between Individual Behaviors and STD Risk?" *Dissertation Abstracts International, A: The Humanities and Social Sciences*, 60, 4, Oct, 1341-A.

Rosenthal, Susan L., Frank M. Biro, Shelia S. Cohen, Paul A. Succop, and Lawrence R. Stanberry. 1995. "Strategies for Coping with Sexually

Transmitted Diseases by Adolescent Females." *Adolescence,* 30, 119:655–66.

Rupp, R., Rosenthal, S., and L. Stanberry. 2005. "Pediatrics and herpes simplex virus vaccines." *Seminars in Pediatric Infectious Diseases,* 16, 1:31–37

Sandelowski, Margarete, Lambe, Camille, and Julie Barroso. 2004. "Stigma in HIV-Positive Women." *Journal of Nursing Scholarship,* 36, 2: 122–128.

Sandstrom, Kent L. 1990. "Confronting Deadly Disease: The Drama of Identity Construction among Gay Men with AIDS." *Journal of Contemporary Ethnography,* 19, 3:271–94.

———. 1996. "Redefining Sex and Intimacy: The Sexual Self-Images, Outlooks, and Relationships of Gay Men Living with HIV/AIDS." *Symbolic Interaction* 19:241–62.

———. 1998. "Preserving a Vital and Valued Self in the Face of AIDS." *Sociological Inquiry,* 68, 3:354–71.

Sanger-Katz, Margot. Jan. 7, 2007. "Demand high for HPV shot: Doctor's offices say supplies are limited." *Concord Monitor.* Retrieved, May 31, 2007, from http://www.concordmonitor.com.

Sarbin, Theodore R. 1986. "The narrative as a root metaphor for psychology." In T.R. Sarbin (ed.) *Narrative psychology: The storied nature of human conduct,* pp. 3–21. New York: Praeger.

Schneider, Joseph W. and Peter Conrad. 1981. "In the Closet with Illness: Epilepsy, Stigma Potential and Information Control." *Social Problems,* 28, 1:32–44

Schwartz, Michael, G.F.N. Fearn, and Sheldon Stryker. 1966. "A note on self conception and the emotionally disturbed role." Sociometry, 29:300–05.

Seeff, L.C. and M.T. McKenna. 2003. "Cervical cancer mortality among foreign-born women living in the United States, 1985 to 1996." *Cancer Detection & Prevention* 27: 203–208.

Shrier, Lydia A., Elizabeth Goodman, and S. Jean Emans. 1999. "Partner Condom Use among Adolescent Girls with Sexually Transmitted Diseases." *Journal of Adolescent Health,* 1999, 24, 5:357–61.

Signorielli, Nancy. 1993. *Mass Media Images and the Impact on Health: A Sourcebook.* Wesport, CT: Greenwood Press.

Smoak, N.D. Scott-Sheldon, L.A., Johnson, B.T., and M.P. Carey. 2006. "Sexual risk reduction interventions do not inadvertently increase the overall frequency of sexual behavior: a meta-analysis of 174 studies with 116,735 participants." *Journal of Acquired Immune Deficiency Syndrome* 41: 374–84.

Smyth, Deidre M. 1998. Common Sense Understanding of the Female Alcoholic, *Annual Meeting of the Society for the Study of Social Problems*: San Francisco, CA.

Spiro, David and Fred Heidrich. 1983. Lay Understanding of Medical Terminology, *The Journal of Family Practice*, 17:277–9.

Strauss, Anselm L. 1959. *Mirrors and Masks*. Mill Valley, CA: Sociology Press.

Swanson, Janice M., and W. Carole Chenitz. 1993. "Regaining a Valued Self: The Process of Adaptation to Living with Genital Herpes." *Qualitative Health Research*, 3, 3:270–97.

Summers, Ann. 1975. *Damned Whores and God's Police: the Colonization of Women in Australia*. Melbourne, Australia: Penguin Books.

Temte, Jonathan L. 2007. "HPV Vaccine: A Cornerstone of Female Health." *American Family Physician*, 75, 1: 28–30.

Tewksbury, Richard, and Deanna McGaughey. 1997. "Stigmatization of Persons with HIV Disease: Perceptions, Management and Consequences of AIDS." *Sociological Spectrum*, 17:49–70.

Thomas, James C., Michele Clark, Jadis Robinson, Martha Monnett, Peter H. Kilmarx, and Thomas A. Peterman. 1999. "The Social Ecology of Syphilis." *Social Science & Medicine*, 48, 8:1081–94.

Thomson, Rachel. 1994. "Moral Rhetoric and Public Health Pragmatism: The Recent Politics of Sex Education." *Feminist Review*, 48:40–60.

Thomson, Rachel and Holland, Janet. 1994. 'Young Women and Safer (Hetero)Sex: Context, Constraints and Strategies', in Sue Wilkinson and Celia Kitzinger (eds.) *Women and Health: Feminist Perspectives*, pp. 13–32. London: Taylor & Francis.

Waitzkin, Howard. 1989. "A Critical Theory of Medical Discourse: Ideology, Social Control, and the Processing of Social Context in Medical Encounters." *Journal of Health and Social Behavior*, 30:220–39.

———. 1991. *The Politics of Medical Encounters: How Patients and Doctors Deal with Social Problems*. New Haven, CT: Yale University Press.

Waller, Jo, McCaffery, Kirsten, Forrest, Sue, and Jane Wardle. 2004. "Human Papillomavirus and Cervical Cancer: Issues for Biobehavioral and Psychosocial Research." *Annals of Behavioral Medicine*, 27, 1:68–79.

Walby, Syliva. 1990. *Theorizing Patriarchy*. Oxford: Basil Blackwell.

Weinstock, H., Berman, S., and W. Cates, Jr. 2004. "Sexually Transmitted Diseases among American Youth: Incidence and Prevalence Estimates, 2000." *Perspectives on Sexual and Reproductive Health*, 36, 1: 6–10.

Weitz, Rose. 1991. *Life with AIDS*. New Brunswick, NJ: Rutgers University Press.

Wiseman, Jacqueline P. 1970. *Stations of the Lost*. Chicago: University of Chicago Press.

Woolley, F. Ross, Kane, Robert L., Hughes, Charles C. and Diana D. Wright. 1978. "The Effects of Doctor-Patient Communication on Satisfaction and Outcome of Care." *Social Science & Medicine*, 12:123–28.

World Health Organization. 2007. "Vaccinating Against Cervical Cancer." *Bulletin of the World Health Organization*. 85, 2: 89–90.

Zimet GD. 2006. "Understanding and overcoming barriers to human Papillomavirus vaccine acceptance." Current Opinion in Obstetric Gynecology. 18, 1:S23–28.

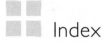

Index

Adina Nack is Associate Professor of Sociology at California Lutheran University and has been involved with sexual health education for more than a decade as an outreach worker, health educator, researcher, as well as a professor of sexuality studies. She is a member of Ventura County's HIV/AIDS Coalition and, for several years has been the organizer of the county's World AIDS Day events. Visit her website at www.adinanack.com